Simple Steps
to a Healthier Lifestyle

as revealed by science

By

Celia M. Ross, M.S.

See your physician regularly and discuss any changes you plan to make to your health program with him/her.

ISBN 0-7414-2327-8

Published by:

INFINITY
PUBLISHING.COM

1094 New De Haven Street, Suite 100
West Conshohocken, PA 19428-2713
Info@buybooksontheweb.com
www.buybooksontheweb.com
Toll-free (877) BUY BOOK
Local Phone (610) 941-9999
Fax (610) 941-9959

Printed in the United States of America

Printed on Recycled Paper

Published March 2005

To the memory of my mother,
Sophie Ross.

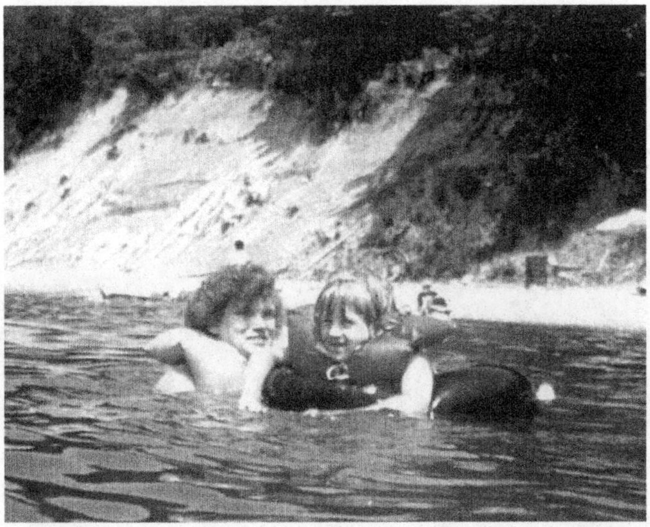

Special thanks to:

Bill Bray Writers' Group,
Winston-Salem, NC
braymoderator@yahoo.com

Morgan Turner
Artist
Morgan_Tami@bellsouth.net

Introduction

Too busy to follow an intensive health program and cook the prescribed gourmet meals three times a day?

From researching databases of medical literature, I've uncovered simple things you can do to improve your health. Many don't take a lot of time. For example, did you know that snacking on nuts can cut your risk of coronary heart disease by 30-50%, or that magnesium supplementation can reduce your risk of developing type 2 diabetes?

You choose whichever suggestions are right for you. Are you concerned about a family history of cancer? There's a chapter on cancer. Has your doctor told you that you are at risk for heart disease? I've included a chapter about the heart. Many of the suggestions take just a few minutes a day.

Satisfy your inner child who always asks "why?" Not only does this book provide practical health-hints, I also offer brief, plain-spoken explanations about the research behind them.

Concerned about the health of a loved one?

Simple steps to a healthier lifestyle is a fun and interesting read, making it a great gift item.

Bone

Jump around!

Jumping rope isn't just for kids – it's a great way to strengthen bones.

Not coordinated enough to jump rope?

No need to use the rope. Just turn on some music and jump to it.

Don't have the stamina to jump around for long periods of time?

No problem. Research on *osteogenic* – bone building – response to stimuli, indicates that multiple short bursts of exercise per day might be better than a single long dose.

What about running? Or walking for that matter?

Walking and running are good bone strengthening exercises. However, on rainy days you might try jumping indoors. Research on rats indicates that jumping is more effective than running for strengthening the bones.

Here's the science:

Medical researchers in Japan trained rats to jump. They found that eight weeks of jump training improved various parameters of leg bone (tibia) strength.

Researchers at the University of Arizona tested jump-rope training on high school girls. They found that 10 minutes a day of jump-rope training for 4 months had a positive effect on leg (femur) and lower back (lumbar spine) strength (BMI, OCSI).

Med Sci Sports Exerc. 2002 Dec; 34(12): 1913-9.
J Bone Miner Res. 2001 Sep; 16(9): 1688-93.
J Bone Miner Res. 2000 Aug; 15(8): 1596-602.
Int J Sports Med. 1995 Aug; 16(6): 364-7.

B$_{12}$ones.

Don't eat a lot of animal products (meat, eggs, milk)? You could be at high risk for osteoporosis.

If you're a vegetarian or nearly so, take daily B$_{12}$ or multivitamin supplements.

Here's the science:

Vitamin B$_{12}$, which is found in animal products, is important for bone health. A study of senior women found that those with the lowest B$_{12}$ levels had greater bone loss as measured by bone mineral density (BMD).

B$_{12}$ones

http://www.eurekalert.org/pub_releases/2004-03/es-vbl030304.php

Bone

Eat green.

For strong bones, include lots of dark green, leafy vegetables in your balanced diet. For insurance, take a multivitamin.

Here's the science:

Bone tissue is more than just mineral. Its strength also depends on collagen cross-linking. Collagen is a major protein of the extracellular matrix – the mortar that holds the cells together. Collagen is a fiberous protein that forms a mesh network, which helps give bone its strength.

Homocysteine is a toxic, metabolic by-product. High homocysteine levels impede collagen cross-linking in bone tissue. In the Framingham Study, high homocysteine levels were associated with greater hip fracture rates.

B-complex, especially folate, suppresses homocysteine levels thereby enabling normal collagen crossing-linking. Folate is found in dark green leafy vegetables. To make sure you get all your B vitamins every day, take a multivitamin.

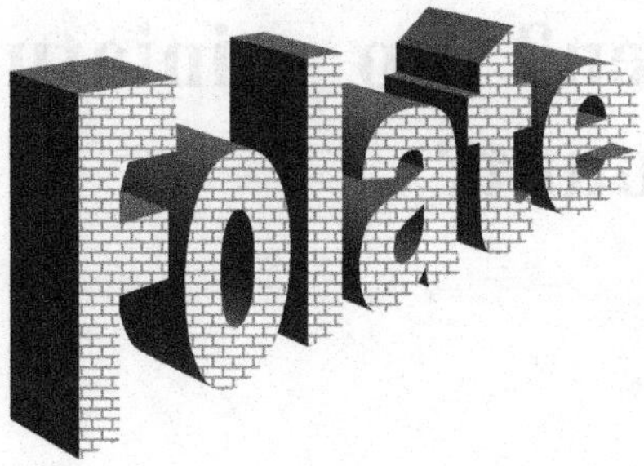

---

http://content.nejm.org/cgi/content/abstract/350/20/2042
http://www.nature.com/cgi-taf/DynaPage.taf?file=/ejcn/journal/v58/n2/abs/1601795a.html

Bone

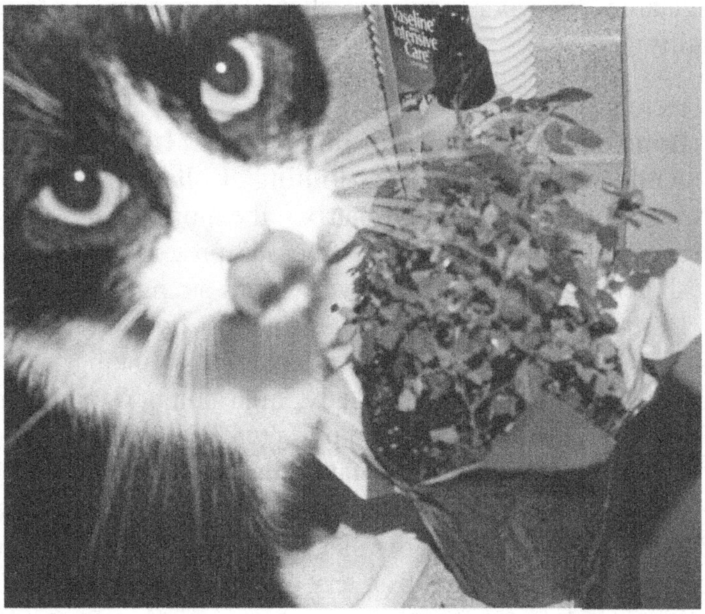

Eat green? Do miniature rose leaves count?

Bone

Don't let stress break you (or your bones).

Calm down. Stress weakens your bones.

Simplify your life. What changes can you make to reduce negative stress?

Take fish oil supplements. Fish oil suppresses stress-induced increases in the hormone cortisol. Use pharmaceutical-grade fish oil to avoid contaminants.

Take a hike. Exercise training helps to lower basal cortisol levels.

Here's the science:

Chronic stress results in the increased release of cortisol into the blood. High cortisol levels suppresses the function of cells (osteoblasts) that build bone tissue and activates cells (osteoclasts) that eat-away at bones. This can lead to osteoporosis.

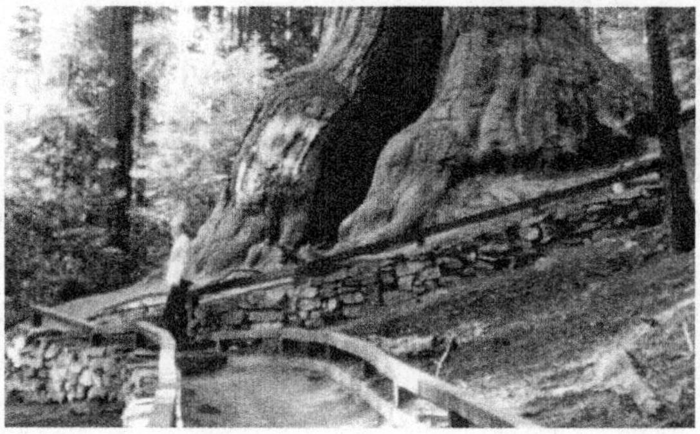

Go for a walk in the woods.

---

http://www.e2med.com/index.cfm?fuseaction=viewArtDossier&DartIdx=151325&DIssIdx=8801&DChapIdx=66135
Chin J Physiol. 2001 Mar 31;44(1):13-8.
Coll Antropol. 2001 Dec;25(2):485-92.
http://www.blackwell-synergy.com/openurl?genre=article&sid=nlm:pubmed&issn=0002-8614&date=2001&volume=49&issue=6&spage=732
Trends Endocrinol Metab. 2001 Jul;12(5):198-203.
http://www.eurekalert.org/pub_releases/1999-08/ACS-SsvC-220899.php

Bone

Build some backbone.

Vertebral fractures are a painful consequence of osteoporosis. However, resistance exercises that tone your back muscles, strengthen your backbone as well. Ask the trainer at your fitness center to show you how to do the following:

Shrugs (neck) – while holding a pair of dumbbells, slowly shrug your shoulders.

Rowing machine (upper back) – you can also row using a dumbbell.

Lat pull-down machine (middle back) – it exercises the same muscles as pull-ups (chinning), but you can use a lot less weight.

Lumbar extensor machine (lower back) – it exercises the same muscles as the Roman chair but you can use less weight.

Here's the science:

Exercise strengthens bones around the site where the muscles attach to the bone. Just as muscles adapt to an increased workload, the skeleton remodels to adjust to increased demands. By looking at a skeleton, scientists can tell what muscles the person used the most. Three-thousand years from now, archaeologists will be able to guess whether you were a couch potato or not.

---

http://www.transplantjournal.com/pt/re/transplantation/abstract.00007890-200308150-00019.htm
Larsen, C.S. Bioarchaeology. 1997

Bone

Have a piece of fruit with that cheese.

Everyone knows that calcium is important for building bones, but did you know that certain fruits and berries aid bone strength, too?

To ward off osteoporosis have some strawberries or apple slices with your cheese (or calcium supplement). Then wash it down with purple grape juice.

Here's the science:

The *phytochemical* – plant chemical – quercetin helps to keep bones from dissolving away. Osteoclasts are cells that take-away calcium from bones, causing the formation of microscopic pits in the bones. Quercetin inhibits osteoclasts. It works in two ways:

Quercetin keeps your baby osteoclasts (osteoclast progenitor cells) from turning into bone-munching machines. Quercetin inhibits the activation of two transcription factors – molecular hands that flip genetic switches – involved in the maturation of osteoclasts.

Quercetin suppresses the bone-eating activity of mature osteoclasts.

This important phytochemical is found in various fruits and berries, including apples, mangos, strawberries, cranberries, and grapes.

---

http://www.sciencedirect.com/science?_ob=ArticleURL&_udi=B6T4P-473MFG5-1&_coverDate=01%2F01%2F2003&_alid=169116770&_rdoc=1&_fmt=&_orig=search&_qd=1&_cdi=4980&_sort=d&view=c&_acct=C000050221&_version=1&_urlVersion=0&_userid=10&md5=739311ab66642fcd2611d68e90d3e0c0

http://www.jstage.jst.go.jp/article/bpb/27/4/27_504/_article

http://www3.interscience.wiley.com/cgi-bin/abstract/108061346/ABSTRACT

Biogerontology. 2002;3(1-2):79-83.

J Agric Food Chem. 2004 Jan 28;52(2):188-95

J Agric Food Chem. 2004 Mar 24;52(6):1586-9

J Agric Food Chem. 2004 Mar 10;52(5):1281-6

Bone

A-soy – there, matey!

One in four women over age 65 has osteoporosis. Many end up suffering painful fractures. Their condition often forces them into nursing homes. If you are a woman over 45, put some soy in your diet to help keep your bones strong.

Drink soy milk. Chocolate soy milk tastes great.
Snack on soy nuts. They are high in protein, too.
Use soy milk instead of regular milk in your favorite recipes.
Try tofu.

Here's the science:
Soy isoflavones – a class of phytochemicals – have a beneficial effect on the bone mass of perimenopausal and postmenopausal women. Soy isoflavones do this because they are *selective estrogen receptor modulators.* Different tissues contain different types of estrogen receptors. Soy isoflavones have different affinities for these different receptors. Thus, unlike estrogen replacement therapy, soy strengthens a woman's bones without increasing her breast cancer risk.

---

http://www.eurekalert.org/pub_releases/2002-06/uoc--oic061002.php
http://jcem.endojournals.org/cgi/content/abstract/88/10/4740
http://www.eurekalert.org/pub_releases/2000-08/AJoC-Ispm-2708100.php
http://www.jacn.org/cgi/content/full/20/suppl_5/354S

Tofu Salad

14 oz. block of light tofu
2 cups leaf Romaine or Ruby lettuce
1½ cups baby spinach
1 cup shredded red cabbage
1 cup shredded carrot
1 red bell pepper, sliced
7 tablespoons balsamic vinegar
4 tablespoons extra-virgin olive oil
2 tablespoons fresh rosemary leaves
1 tablespoon oregano

Cut tofu into bite-sized pieces. Place tofu in a zipper-type plastic bag. Add spices and 3 tablespoons of balsamic vinegar. Close bag. Toss. Refrigerate overnight.

Prepare salad. Toss. Portion out onto plates. Add tofu. Serve. Drizzle with extra-virgin olive oil and balsamic vinegar. Eat.

Yield: serves two.

Cancer

A berry good idea.

Chop up some fruit and have a fresh fruit and berry salad.

Here's the science:

The *phytochemicals* – plant chemicals – found in fruits and berries work together to attack cancer from different angles.

Bananas reduce colorectal cancer risk.

Blueberries have high antioxidant activity. They detoxify highly reactive chemicals called free radicals. Left unchecked, free radicals damage DNA, causing mutations, some of which can lead to cancer.

Raspberry and blueberry extracts prevent damage to DNA by carcinogens, damage which could lead to cancer.

Citrus fruits contain phytochemicals that inhibit cancer cells proliferation. Two phytochemicals found in tangerines are particularly effective at inhibiting prostate cancer cells. Another one found in oranges and tangerines, inhibits lung cancer cells.

Apple peel extracts inhibit cancer cell proliferation.

Various berry extracts have been found to inhibit the process by which cancer tumors grow new blood vessels. Tumors can't grow if they don't grow more blood vessels.

Pineapples contain the phytochemical bromelain, which has been found to curb the spread (metastasis) of lung cancer.

Am J Clin Nutr. 2003 Sep;78(3 Suppl):517S-520S.
Nutr Cancer. 1996;25(3):297-304.
J Med Food. 2001 Spring;4(1):49-51.
Free Radic Res. 2002 Sep; 36(9): 1023-31.
http://www.eurekalert.org/pub_releases/2000-03/ACS-Nsio-2003100.php
http://www.jbc.org/cgi/content/abstract/279/11/10670
http://www.eurekalert.org/pub_releases/2000-06/CUNS-Apfc-2006100.php
J Cancer Res Clin Oncol. 1988;114(5):507-8.
Cell Mol Life Sci. 2001 Aug;58(9):1234-45

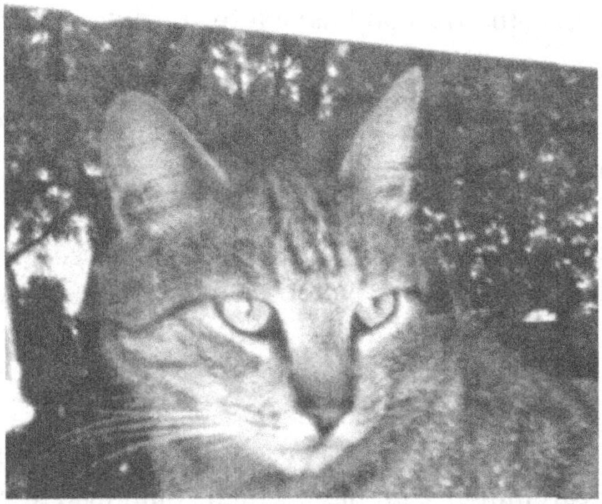

Free radicals? You mean like tiny anarchists inside my body, turning over cars and wrecking stuff? I'm glad antioxidants can cuff the bastards.

Cancer

Bottoms up.

Don't just sip your water – drink it! Drinking plenty of water (or green tea) lowers your risk of bladder cancer.

Here's the science:

Greater fluid intake dilutes carcinogens and increases the frequency of voiding. This reduces the contact between carcinogens and the bladder.

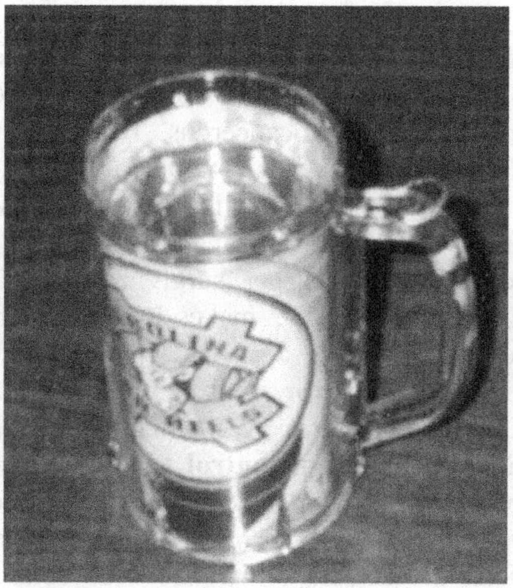

http://content.nejm.org/cgi/content/abstract/340/18/1390

Cancer

Swimming against the tide of cancer.

Take a *pharmaceutical-grade* – purified – fish oil supplement daily. Use the pharmaceutical-grade fish oil supplements to avoid the risk of contamination by pollutants. You can get them at your health food store or at http://nordicnaturals.com.

Here's the science:

Fish oil reduces cancer risk. Both human population and animal studies show that consumption of omega-3 fatty acids found in fish oil protects against cancer.

Omega-3 fatty acids assist cancer cells in committing suicide. Cells are programmed to commit suicide (apoptosis) when they start to turn cancerous. However, sometimes cancer cells override this program. One of the ways that they do this is by using a protein called survivin. Survivin binds to and neutralizes a suicide enzyme.

How do cancer cells get survivin? COX-2 is over-expressed in cancer. COX-2 makes PGE2, which increases survivin levels.

If COX-2 is over-expressed in cancer, how can you regulate COX-2? One way is with omega-3 fatty acids.

Fish oil reigns in out of control AP-1. AP-1 is composed of a pair of proteins. It works like a pair of chopsticks to grab DNA switch sites and turn on genes involved in cell proliferation. In cancer, AP-1 becomes *constitutively* – constantly – *active*. Thus, the cancer cells proliferate uncontrollably. The omega-3 fatty acid DHA helps keep AP-1 from going out of control.

---

http://www.pnas.org/cgi/content/full/98/13/7510
http://www.nutrition.org/cgi/content/full/132/11/3508S
Cancer Res. 2004 Sep 15;64(18):6359-6362
World J Gastroenterol. 2004 Sep 15;10(18):2759-61.
FASEB J. 2004 Jan;18(1):206-8.

Cancer

Play it again!

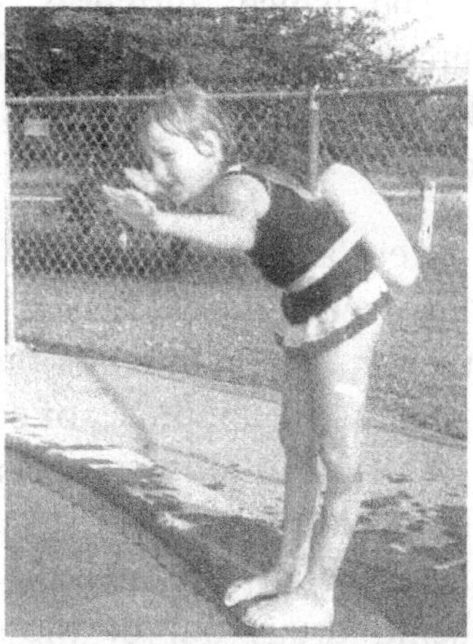

Vigorous play isn't just for children. What did you like doing as a child? Swimming? Dancing? Play it again and exercise your way to a lower cancer risk.

Here's the science:

Exercise reduces breast cancer risk. Thirty to sixty minutes a day of moderate-to-vigorous exercise reduces breast cancer risk by 20-30%.

Exercise reduces colon cancer risk. Thirty to sixty minutes a day of moderate-to-vigorous activity reduces colon cancer risk.

Several mechanisms are involved.

Moderate-to-vigorous physical activity balances female hormone levels. This may help reduce breast cancer risk.

Exercise initiates a series of biochemical reactions that regulate an enzyme involved in cell growth (mTOR). Inappropriate cell growth is a key step in the development of cancer.

Physical activity reduces the risk of developing type 2 diabetes, a risk factor for cancer. The high insulin levels found in type 2 diabetes stimulate cancer cell growth. High blood sugar may be another contributing factor. High blood sugar depletes antioxidants. With the antioxidant shield down, DNA is more vulnerable to attack by free radicals.

---

http://care.diabetesjournals.org/cgi/content/full/26/6/1752
http://content.nejm.org/cgi/content/abstract/336/18/1269
http://www.acsm-msse.org/pt/re/msse/abstract.00005768-200311000-00007.htm
J Natl Cancer Inst. 1999 Aug 4;91(15):1334.
New Scientist 2004 Aug 14 183(2460):34-37.

Cancer

Get spicy.

The spice turmeric contains phytochemicals called curcuminoids, which have anti-cancer properties. If you don't like spicy food, curcuminoids are available in capsule form.

Here's the science:

Curcuminoids assist cancer cells in committing suicide. Curcuminoids reduce COX-2 expression thus encouraging apoptosis of cancer cells.

Curcuminoids increase tumors' sensitivity to chemotherapy. Some cancer tumors develop resistance to chemotherapy by making a bunch of pumps that pump chemo drugs out of the cell. Curcuminoids decrease the cancer cells' production of them.

---

http://carcin.oupjournals.org/cgi/content/abstract/24/9/1515
http://www.sciencedirect.com/science?_ob=ArticleURL&_udi=B6T2D-4B959HX-3&_coverDate=02%2F14%2F2004&_alid=168306847&_rdoc=1&_fmt=&_orig=search&_qd=1&_cdi=4916&_sort=d&view=c&_acct=C000050221&_version=1&_urlVersion=0&_userid=10&md5=853350b9961dd52af417fa83171b7cf7
http://www.biomedcentral.com/1471-2407/4/13
Cancer Res. 2004 Sep 15;64(18):6359-6362
World J Gastroenterol. 2004 Sep 15;10(18):2759-61.

Cancer

<u>Spicy Potato</u>

1 cooked, cold potato, peeled and diced
1 red bell pepper, cut into bite-sized pieces
2 tablespoon canola oil
1 teaspoon turmeric
2 teaspoons paprika
1 teaspoon coarse ground black pepper
2 tablespoon freeze-dried chives

Preheat frying pan and oil, medium heat. In a bowl, toss diced potato and spices until the potato pieces are covered with spice. Add red bell pepper. Pour into frying pan. Stir while cooking for about 12 minutes. Serve.

Yield: serves two.

Cancer

Not only for your heart…

Are you taking aspirin for your heart? You might be warding off cancer too. Aspirin reduces cancer risk by inhibiting COX-2. Concerned about a family history of cancer? Or a recurrence of cancer? Talk to your doctor about aspirin.

Here's the science:

Aspirin decreases cancer risk. It reduces the risk of colorectal cancer by 35%. Aspirin also decreases the risk of breast, prostate, lung, and skin cancer.

COX-2 is over expressed in cancer cells. Excess COX-2 activity helps cancer cells thrive. COX-2 makes the chemical PGE2. PGE2 allows cancer cells to override the suicide program, which normally knocks-out defective cells.

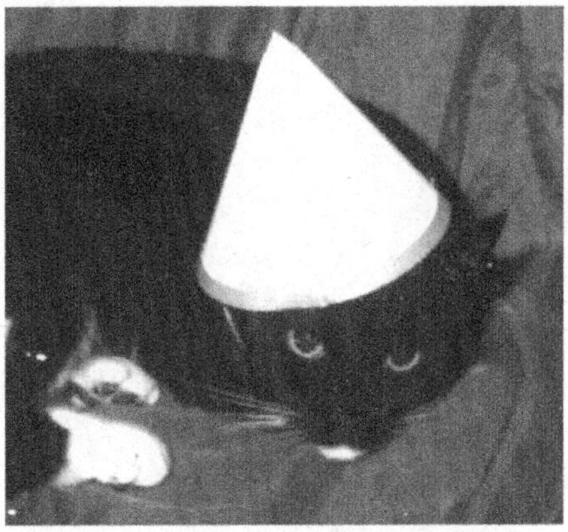

Aspirin isn't just for New Year's Day.

FASEB J. 2004 Jan;18(1):206-8.
Curr Cancer Drug Targets. 2004 Feb;4(1):29-42.
http://www.eurekalert.org/pub_releases/2003-03/dms-aaa030403.php
Cancer Res. 2004 Sep 15;64(18):6359-6362.

Cancer

Want to keep a healthy figure?

The phytochemicals in Concord (purple) grape juice inhibit chemically-induced mammary (breast) cancer in rats. Concord grape juice reduced the number of tumors and the tumor mass.

Here's the science:

Purple grape juice is rich in a variety of anticancer phytochemicals.

Antioxidants found in grape juice helps protect DNA from damage by free radicals.

Anti-carcinogenic. Resveratrol, one of the phytochemicals found in grape juice, inhibits DNA damage from a carcinogen.

Modulates gene expression. Quercetin, another grape phytochemical, inhibits the expression of specific oncogenes – cancer genes – while increasing the expression of several tumor suppressor genes.

Assists apoptosis. Quercetin and resveratrol assist cancer cells in committing suicide.

Augments chemo. Quercetin enhances the ability of Cisplatin – a chemo drug – to kill cancer cells.

---

http://www.eurekalert.org/pub_releases/2002-11/ajoc-cgj112002.php
J Agric Food Chem. 2003 Dec 3;51(25):7280-6.
http://www.sciencedirect.com/science?_ob=ArticleURL&_udi=B6T2C-494CJ20-2&_coverDate=08%2F28%2F2003&_alid=175951350&_rdoc=1&_fmt=&_orig=search&_qd=1&_cdi=4915&_sort=d&view=c&_acct=C000050221&_version=1&_urlVersion=0&_userid=10&md5=5699856daa691d8c6cfe1280a006e307
http://cdli.asm.org/cgi/content/abstract/11/1/63
http://carcin.oupjournals.org/cgi/content/full/25/5/647
http://www.nature.com/cgi-taf/DynaPage.taf?file=/bjc/journal/vaop/ncurrent/abs/6601898a.html&dynoptions=doi1086016651
Anticancer Res. 2004 Mar-Apr;24(2B):987-98.
Folia Morphol (Warsz). 2004 Feb;63(1):103-5.

Cancer

Orange you a smart bunny.

Carrots contain a variety of carotenoids – orange colored phytochemicals that fight cancer. Other sources of carotenoids include tomatoes, sweet potatoes, yams, oranges, red bell peppers, spinach and other dark greens (the green conceals the orange pigment – think about leaves in the fall).

Here's the science:

Carotenoids act as antioxidants. The slight differences in the structure of assorted carotenoids mean that they partition differently within cells – protecting separate sections of the cell (lipid membrane versus watery parts) from free radicals.

Carotenoids aid immune function. A strong immune system can often kill cancer before it grows into a tumor.

Carotenoids improve cellular communication. Carontenoids, especially lycopene, help cells talk to one another. A breakdown in cell-cell communication plays a role in the development of cancer.

Carrot Salad

4 cups shredded carrots
1 cup raisins or to taste
1 20-oz. can crushed pineapple

Mix. Refrigerate. Eat.

Yield: serves ten.

---

http://www.ajcn.org/cgi/content/full/71/2/575
http://www.ajcn.org/cgi/content/full/72/4/990
Mol Aspects Med. 1993;14(3):241-6.
http://www.nutrition.org/cgi/content/abstract/134/1/257S
http://www.nutrition.org/cgi/content/full/132/12/3754
http://www.nutrition.org/cgi/content/abstract/134/4/935

Cancer

Stuffed Red Bell Peppers

4 red bell peppers
2 baked yams
26 oz. jar of pasta sauce
2 teaspoons oregano
1 teaspoon coarse ground black pepper
1 vegetable burger, diced
3 cups frozen mixed vegetables

Preheat oven to 350 degrees.

Measure out 2 cups pasta sauce, place in bowl. Scoop out 1 cup baked yam. Blend sauce and yam with a fork. Mix in oregano and pepper. Mix in diced vegetable burger. Mix in frozen vegetables.

Remove the tops of the peppers and deseed. Place burger/vegetable mixture in peppers. Place peppers in baking dish. Pour the rest of the pasta sauce into the baking dish. Bake peppers for about 40 minutes.

Yield: serves four.

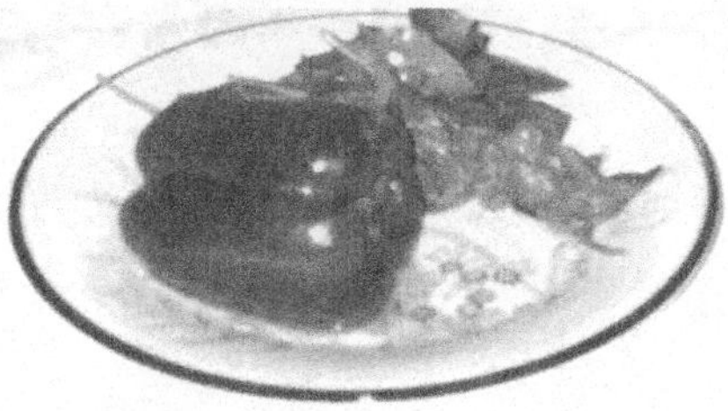

Cancer

Slice of Life

Large tomatoes, sliced thick
Cucumbers, diced
Red onion, diced
Feta cheese crumbles
Extra-virgin olive oil
Balsamic vinegar

Place cucumbers, onion, and feta cheese on top of tomato slices. Drizzle vinegar and olive oil over the slices. Serve.

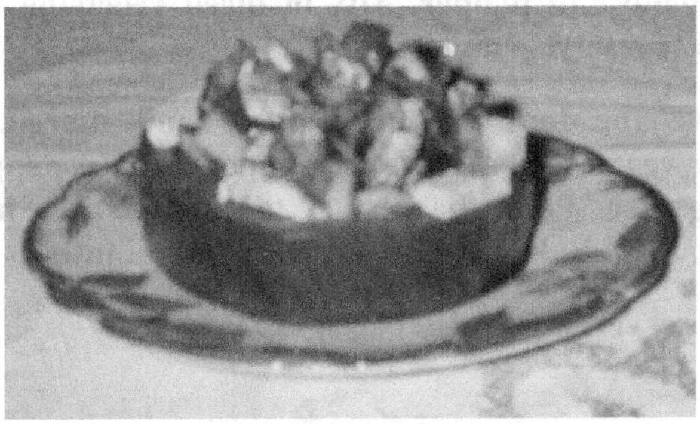

Cancer

The refined cereal killer.

When possible, choose whole grains over refined cereals (white bread, pasta, rice). A high consumption of refined cereals is associated with an increased risk of cancer.

Here's the science:

High blood sugar from eating a lot of high glycemic refined carbohydrates creates reactive oxygen species.

High plasma insulin. A high glycemic index diet triggers compensatory increases in insulin, which can stimulate cancer cell growth.

Lack of fiber. A diet high in refined cereals may lack the fiber found in whole grains, fruits, and vegetables. A low fiber diet increases colon cancer risk.

Lack of phytochemicals. Whole grains contain phytochemicals that refined cereal lacks.

---

http://www.ajcn.org/cgi/content/full/70/6/1107
J Natl Cancer Inst. 1999 Aug 4;91(15):1334.
Am J Clin Nutr. 2004 Feb;79(2):274-81.
http://www.nutrition.org/cgi/content/abstract/134/4/935
J Agric Food Chem. 2003 Dec 17;51(26):7825-34.
http://www.jacn.org/cgi/content/full/19/1/61
http://www.foxnews.com/story/0,2933,130345,00.html

Homeland Hotcakes

1 cup whole wheat flour
½ cup Splenda
2 teaspoon baking powder
½ teaspoon salt
1¼ cups soy milk
¼ cup canola oil
1 cage free egg
1 cup blueberries
1 cup diced strawberries

Mix dry ingredients. Add wet other ingredients. Mix. Add berries. Mix. Pour ½ cup at a time onto a preheated oiled frying pan. Spread out. Flip. Serve. Top with applesauce.

Yield: 6 hotcakes.

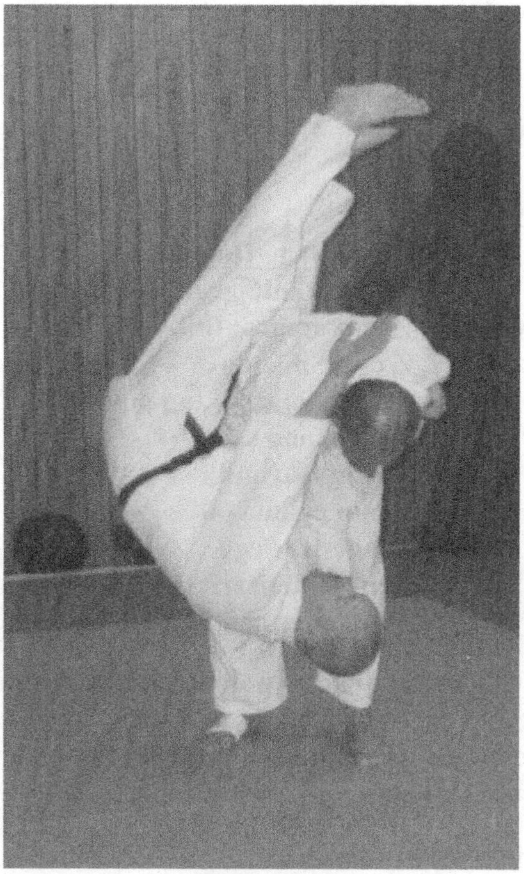

Flip

for whole-grain hotcakes.

Spelt – an ancient cousin of wheat. Farmers grew it 7,000 years ago.

Amaranth – a nutritious seed used by the Aztecs.

Heritage Hotcakes

¾ cup whole-grain spelt flour
¼ cup amaranth flour
½ cup Splenda
2 teaspoons baking powder
½ teaspoon salt
1¼ cup soy milk
¼ cup canola oil
1 cage-free egg
1 cup blueberries
1 cup chopped pecans

Mix flour, Splenda, baking powder, and salt. Blend in soy milk, oil, and egg. Add berries and nuts. Mix. Pour ½ cup at a time onto a preheated oiled frying pan. Spread out. Flip. Serve. Top with applesauce.

Yield: 6 hotcakes.

Cancer

Yummy Yammy Hotcakes

2 yams
1 cup whole wheat flour
½ cup Splenda
2 teaspoons baking powder
½ teaspoon salt
½ teaspoon cinnamon
1¼ cup soy milk
¼ cup canola oil
1 cage-free egg
1 cup chopped pecans

Cook yams at 350 degrees for 1 hour 40 minutes. Let cool. Mix flour, Splenda, baking powder, salt, and cinnamon. Blend in soy milk, oil, and egg. Scoop out yam. Add one cup of yam to batter. Mix well. Add nuts. Mix. Pour ½ cup at a time onto a preheated oiled frying pan. Spread out. Flip. Serve. Top with applesauce.

Yield: 6 hotcakes.

<u>Thanksgiving Day Bread</u>

$^{2}/_{3}$ cup Splenda
2¼ cup whole wheat flour
½ teaspoon salt
1 teaspoon baking soda
2 teaspoons ground cinnamon
$^{1}/_{3}$ cup canola oil
2 cage-free eggs
¾ cup cranberry juice
3 baked yams
1 cup cranberries
½ cup chopped pecans
½ cup chopped dates

Preheat oven to 350 degrees. Mix dry ingredients. Mix in oil, eggs, and cranberry juice. Scoop out 2 cups of yam from the baked yams. Add 2 cups yam to batter, mix well with fork. Mix in cranberries, pecans, and dates. Place in non-stick loaf pan. Bake for about 50 minutes.

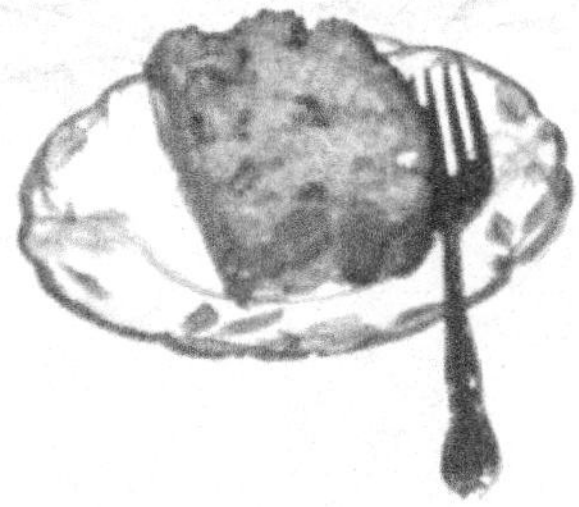

Cancer

Tea time.

Why *green* tea?

Polyphenols. Tea leaves contain a class of phytochemicals called polyphenols. Green tea is made by heating the tea leaves right after harvesting, thus preserving the leaves' natural polyphenols. Black tea, by contrast, is made by crushing and drying the leaves. This gives the leaves time to ferment, which alters their polyphenol mixture. The polyphenol blend in green tea has greater anticancer activity than that of black tea.

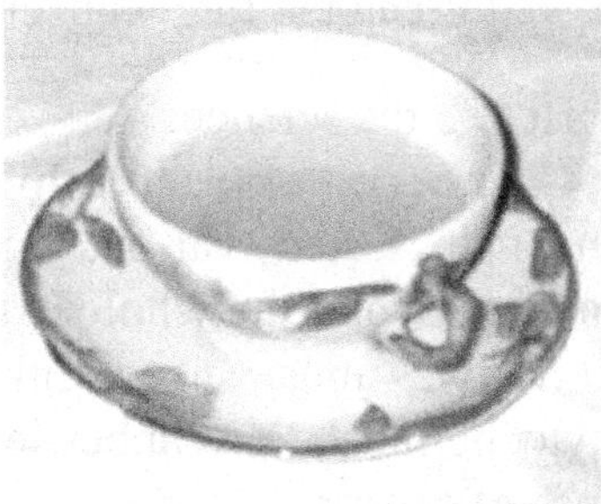

Here's the science:

Green tea polyphenols are antioxidants. In a study comparing the consumption of green tea and black tea, green tea significantly reduced oxidative damage whereas black tea did not.

Green tea polyphenols promote apoptosis (death) of cancer cells.

Green tea polyphenols inhibit tumor growth by repressing new blood vessel development in tumors.

---

http://www.sciencenews.org/articles/20030920/food.asp
In Vivo. 2004 Jan-Feb;18(1):73-80.
http://www.sciencedirect.com/science?_ob=ArticleURL&_udi=B6T99-4BBKH1X-1&_coverDate=02%2F06%2F2004&_alid=176761581&_rdoc=1&_fmt=&_orig=search&_qd=1&_cdi=5109&_sort=d&view=c&_acct=C000050221&_version=1&_urlVersion=0&_userid=10&md5=ebcadad66af776a80c4a1fee4d1461ad
http://www.nutrition.org/cgi/content/abstract/133/10/3303S
http://cancerres.aacrjournals.org/cgi/content/abstract/63/23/8118
http://www3.interscience.wiley.com/cgi-bin/abstract/104541740/ABSTRACT

Cancer

Berry good iced tea.

Try mixing equal amounts of cranberry juice and strong-brewed green tea for a cancer-fighting iced tea blend.

Here's the science:

Cranberry extract inhibits cancer cell proliferation. Scientists tested various individual phytochemicals from cranberries and the whole extract. They found that the whole extract was most successful in inhibiting cancer cells. The phytochemicals in cranberries act together to inhibit various types of cancer.

J Agric Food Chem. 2004 May 5;52(9):2512-7
Barbara Fricke

Cancer

Ginger doesn't treat cancer gingerly.

Try a cup of ginger tea. Make ginger tea using 1 teaspoon grated, fresh ginger per cup water.

Here's the science:

Ginger contains the phytochemicals [6]-gingerol and [6]-paradol.

[6]-gingerol moderates AP-1 activity. AP-1, the chopsticks-like pair of proteins, grasps DNA switch sites for cell proliferation.

[6]-paradol promotes apoptosis of cancer cells. Die, cancer cells, die!

---

http://www.eurekalert.org/pub_releases/2003-10/uom-sdg102303.php
http://cancerres.aacrjournals.org/cgi/content/full/61/3/850

Cancer

Don't let it kill you.

Stress is a killer – it leads to a two-fold increase in the risk for breast cancer. So what can you do?

Gain control. Lack of control over your life is a major source of stress. What's causing you to be stress-out? What can you do to gain some control over it? Would simplifying your life help with credit card debit? Are there steps you could take that would help you get a more enjoyable job? Or would it be better to be a stay-at-home mother? How about starting an exercise program and taking control of your health and fitness?

Exercise is an effective way to deal with stress.

Fish oil supplements contain DHA, an important brain nutrient.

Here's the science:

Stress is carcinogenic. A Swedish study found that women who reported living stressful lives had two-fold the rate of breast cancer five years later. This may be due to changes in immune function or alterations in the neuroendocrine – brain/hormone – axes.

Eur J Cancer Prev. 2003 Oct;12(5):377-81.
http://www.eurekalert.org/pub_releases/1999-10/DUMC-DsEm-231099.php
Diabetes Metab. 2003 Jun;29(3):289-95.
Marmot, Michael. The Status Syndrome, 2004.

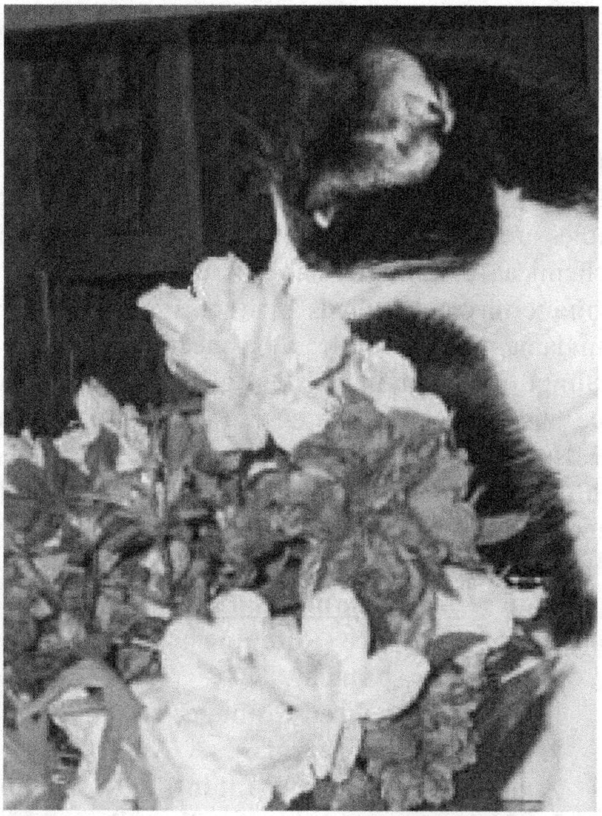

Don't let stress get to you. Take a deep breath and smell the flowers. Then bat your tail for a Tail Chi workout.

Cancer

Cinderella of the vegetable patch.

Cabbage is the Cinderella story of nutrition. It might have a reputation of being peasant food, but it's packed with anti-cancer phytochemicals.

Here's the science:

Cabbage is a cruciferous vegetable. Cruciferous vegetables are rich in chemopreventive – cancer preventing – phytochemicals call indoles and isothiocyanates.

Cabbage phytochemicals protect against free radicals that can damage DNA and lead to cancer.

Cabbage phytochemicals alter gene expression to enhance the cells' own defenses against DNA-damaging chemicals.

Cabbage phytochemicals encourage apoptosis (death) of cancer cells. Thus the cells don't form tumors.

Summer Salad

1 cup leaf lettuce (Romaine or Ruby)
½ cup baby spinach
½ cup shredded red cabbage
½ cup shredded carrot
½ cup red bell pepper, cut into bite-sized pieces
2 tablespoons extra virgin olive oil
1 teaspoon balsamic vinegar

Whisk the olive oil and vinegar together. Pour over salad. Toss. Eat.

Yield: 1 salad.

---

http://cancerres.aacrjournals.org/cgi/content/full/61/16/6120
Integr Cancer Ther. 2004 Mar;3(1):5-12.
http://www.blackwell-synergy.com/openurl?genre=article&sid=nlm:pubmed&issn=1462-8910&date=2004&volume=6&issue=1&spage=28

Digestive

A F.E.W. words about constipation.

You are not alone. Twenty percent of women suffer from constipation. However, it's not something to take lightly. Constipation is associated with more than a two-fold increased risk of colon cancer.

Here's what you can do:

Fiber. Eat lots of fiber-rich fruits and vegetables.

Exercise. Go for a walk.

Water. Drink plenty of fluids.

Here's the science:

Fiber enhances the water content of stools, augments their bulk and increases concentration of short-chain fatty acids in the cecum, all of which promotes colon motility.

Constipation is associated with physical inactivity. Exercise normalizes numerous bodily functions, including digestion.

Drink plenty of water. If it's dried out, it can't slide down the tract.

---

http://www.blackwell-synergy.com/openurl?genre=article&sid=nlm:pubmed&issn=0002-9270&date=2003&volume=98&issue=4&spage=857
http://pediatrics.aappublications.org/cgi/content/full/113/3/e259
Eur J Gastroenterol Hepatol. 2002 Oct;14(10):1053-6.
http://www.jstage.jst.go.jp/article/bbb/66/6/66_1233/_article/-char/en
http://www.gastroenterologynursing.com/pt/re/gastronurse/fulltext.00001610-200201000-00002.htm

Heart

Take heart….

Stress is a risk factor for hardening of the arteries. The type of stress that causes it is not the CEO's stress but rather the soul-destroying hopelessness and lack of control experienced by those at the bottom.

Long term: Are there steps you can take to get a better job? Can you become self-employed?

In the mean time: Take up a sport. Set a 10K race goal and train to achieve it. Join the martial arts and train for competition. Exercise lowers stress and maybe you'll win a gold medal.

Feed your brain with fish oil. DHA, a fatty acid found in fish oil, blunts the stress hormone response.

Here's the science:

Being at the bottom is bad for the heart. Monkeys who are at the bottom of the pecking order are stressed out and get more hardening of the arteries than those on top. This also applies to people. The lower the rank of British civil servants, the lower their level of HDL – good cholesterol – is.

Exercise has anxiety-reducing effects. Research at the University of Illinois at Urbana found that anxiety levels fall after a workout.

Fish oil blunts the effects of stress. Researchers in France found that fish oil supplementation blunts the surges in plasma epinephrine and cortisol that occur during stress.

Marmot, Michael, The Status Syndrome, 2004.
http://atvb.ahajournals.org/cgi/content/full/15/12/2094
Neuroscience. 2004;124(4):985-92.
http://www.eurekalert.org/pub_releases/1997-04/Uola-SBOE-030497.php
http://www.e2med.com/index.cfm?fuseaction=viewArtDossier&DartIdx=151325&DIssIdx=8801&DChapIdx=66135

Go nuts!

Instead of snacking on a donut, try a handful of nuts.

Are you on a low salt diet? No problem. Unsalted nuts are available in the baking aisle of the grocery store.

Here's the science:

Nuts cut heart disease. Frequent nut consumption is associated with a 30-50% decrease in the risk of coronary heart disease.

Almonds, walnuts, pecans, hazelnuts, and macadamia nuts all reduce bad cholesterol (LDL) levels. LDL is often called "bad cholesterol" because it can enter the arterial wall, putting you on the path toward cardiovascular disease.

Nuts are a good source of vitamin E, a potent antioxidant. When LDL in the arterial wall becomes oxidized, it causes arterial cells to secrete a substance that attracts white blood cells. The white blood cells gobble up the oxidized LDL and become bloated foam cells, which are associated with fatty streak lesions.

Nuts are high in arginine, which is used by the body to make nitric oxide (NO). Fatty streaks become fibrous plaques when smooth muscle cells proliferate in the lesion. NO inhibits smooth muscle cell proliferation. NO is also a *vasodilator*, opening up the blood vessels and allowing more blood to flow through.

---

http://www.ebmonline.org/cgi/content/full/222/3/196
J Nutr. 2003 Apr;133(4):1060-3.
J Am Diet Assoc. 2000 Mar;100(3):312-8.
Curr Atheroscler Rep. 1999 Nov;1(3):204-9.
Clin Cardiol. 1999 Jul;22(7 Suppl):III11-5.
Am J Clin Nutr. 1994 May;59(5):995-9.

Smart Cookies

1 cup whole wheat flour
½ cup flaxseed meal
1 teaspoon baking soda
1 teaspoon salt
1 cup almond butter
½ cup canola oil
2½ cups Splenda
2 teaspoons vanilla extract
4 cage-free eggs
1 cup dried cranberries
1 cup currents

Preheat oven to 375 degrees.

In a medium bowl mix flour, flaxseed meal, baking soda, and salt. Put aside.

In a large mixing bowl combine almond butter, oil, Splenda, vanilla extract, and eggs. Mix well. Slowly beat in flour mixture. Mix in cranberries and currents.

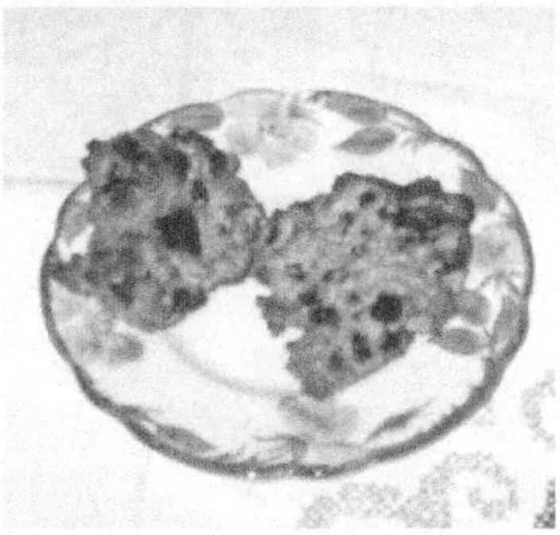

Drop rounded tablespoon fulls of dough onto oiled cookie pan. Bake for about 9 minutes.

Yield: 2 dozen.

Heart

Terrific twosome.

Two antioxidants that form a powerful team to fight hardening of the arteries are vitamin E and coenzyme Q 10. You can get sufficient amounts of vitamin E by eating nuts and whole grains and taking a multivitamin supplement. Coenzyme Q 10 supplements (10 MG) are available at your local health food store.

Here's the science:

Vitamin E and coenzyme Q 10 work better together. In an Australian study done on a breed of mice prone to hardening of the arteries, the two supplements worked better together than either alone in preventing the disease.

Oxidation of LDL is a key step in the formation of hardening of the arteries. Vitamin E and coenzyme Q 10 team-up together to prevent LDL oxidation.

---

http://atvb.ahajournals.org/cgi/content/full/21/4/585

The heart of the big apple.

Apples make a hearty snack. Try these suggestions:

Instead of eating junky snack foods, have an apple. Apples are a convenient nibble.

Replace pancake syrup with applesauce and try putting some oat flour in the pancakes for a healthier breakfast

Add an apple to oatmeal. Dice-up an apple and add it to oatmeal for a heart-healthy meal!

Here's the science:

Apples and oats contain water-soluble fiber. Water-soluble fiber lowers cholesterol levels, decreasing the risk of cardiovascular disease.

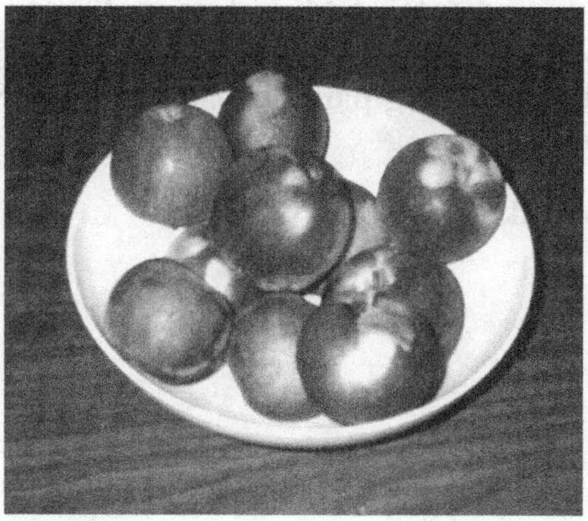

http://circ-meeting.ahajournals.org/cgi/content/abstract/103/9/1366-c
http://www.eurekalert.org/pub_releases/2004-02/jaaj-fif021804.php

Heart

The Big Apple Hotcakes

¾ cup whole wheat flour
¼ cup oat flour
½ cup Splenda
2 teaspoons baking powder
½ teaspoon salt
1 teaspoon cinnamon
1¼ cup soy milk
¼ cup canola oil
1 cage-free egg
2 apples, diced
1 cup chopped pecans

Mix dry ingredients. Add wet ingredients. Mix. Add diced apples and nuts. Mix. Pour ½ cup at a time onto a preheated oiled frying pan. Spread out. Flip. Serve. Top with applesauce.

Yield: 6 hotcakes.

Don't get inflamed when I tell you to watch your weight.

Put on those walking shoes and drop some weight.

Here's the science:

Obesity generates inflammation.

Fat cells make inflammatory molecules (cytokines). The fatter someone is the more inflammatory cytokines their fat cells produce. These cytokines enter the bloodstream.

White blood cells in fatty tissue make inflammatory compounds too. As someone becomes obese, a few fat cells become over-bloated and leak. White blood cells move in to clean up the mess. They then release an inflammatory call for backups.

Obesity increases the risk of developing diabetes. High blood sugar modifies proteins forming *advanced glycation end products* (AGE). AGE-modified proteins trigger an inflammatory response.

Fatty tissue stimulates the production of VLDL. VLDL can trigger an inflammatory response in the arteries.

Inflammation promotes cardiovascular disease.

Inflamed arteries express molecules on their inner surface that cause white blood cells to stick to it. White blood cells then enter the arterial wall. They gobble up any oxidized LDL – bad cholesterol – in the wall and become bloated foam cells. This forms a fatty streak lesion.

Inflammation stimulates smooth muscle cells. Smooth muscle cells move into the lesion and multiply, turning it into a fibrous plaque.

Inflammatory molecules induce foam cells to release enzymes that weaken the fibrous plaque. Debris from disruption of the plaque and thrombosis can lead to a heart attack or stroke.

---

http://circ.ahajournals.org/cgi/content/full/105/9/1135
Science News.2004 165(9):139-140.

Aspirin – the new vitamin?

There's speculation that aspirin should be classified as a vitamin. Aspirin belongs to a group of chemicals called *salicylates*. Salicylates are found in trace amounts in many plants. Our Stone-Age ancestors ate a diet rich in wild fruits and vegetables and thus got a daily dose of these compounds.

Willow bark, which is high in salicylates, was a traditional medicine for fever.

In 1899, the German pharmaceutical firm Bayer patented aspirin. It became a popular medicine for fevers and pain.

In recent years, low-dose aspirin has been recommended for heart health.

Here's the science:

Aspirin and other salicylates work by inhibiting the COX class of enzymes.

Aspirin alleviates pain and inflammation by inhibiting COX-2. This provides aspirin's traditional pain-reliever effect. Recently, inflammation has also been found to play a key role in cardiovascular disease.

By inhibiting COX-1, aspirin reduces the stickiness of platelets, thus preventing the formation of blood clots that could trigger a heart attack. Low-dose aspirin reduces the risk of heart attacks by one-third.

New Scientist. 2004 Feb 07;181(2433):36.

Heart

Take a hike.

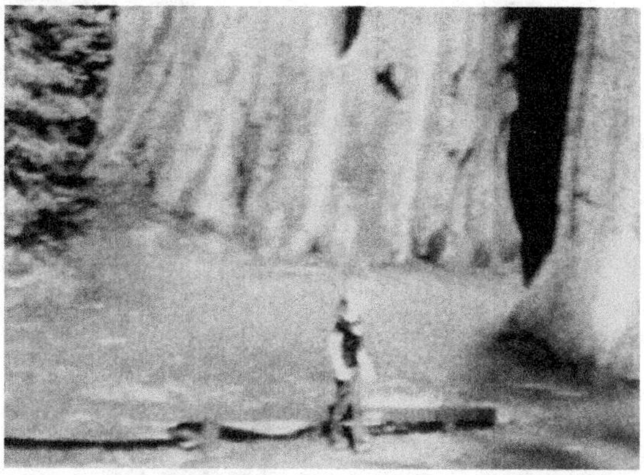

Take brisk daily walks of 20 minutes or more. If you can't walk for 20 minutes, start out with shorter walks and work your way up.

Here's the science:

Walkers show improved blood lipid profiles.

Brisk walking gives you a natural by-pass. Cardiovascular (endurance) exercise encourages the growth of new blood vessels in the heart muscle.

Brisk walking is good for the inner lining of the blood vessels. Nitric oxide (NO) is produced by the cells lining the inner surface of blood vessels (endothelium) in response to exercise. It helps to maintain the health of the vessels.

Cardiovascular exercise reduces the risk of developing Type 2 diabetes. High blood sugar modifies proteins forming *advanced glycation end products* (AGE). AGE-modified proteins trigger an inflammatory response. Inflammation is a risk factor for cardiovascular disease.

---

http://circ.ahajournals.org/cgi/content/full/104/12/1393
http://www.eurekalert.org/pub_releases/2003-08/mc-mcs081503.php
New Scientist.2000 Jan 08;165(2220):10
N Engl J Med. 1999 Aug 26;341(9):650-8.
http://circ.ahajournals.org/cgi/content/full/105/9/1135

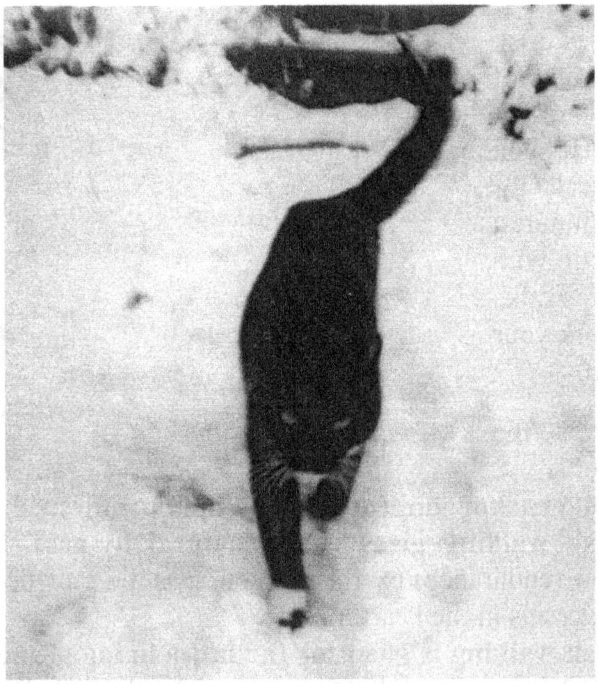

Go for a walk or something – be paws-on about your health.

Heart

A new reason to brush and floss your teeth. (Like you need another?!)

Good dental hygiene does more than give you a beautiful smile. It can help your heart.

Here's the science:

Gum (periodontal) disease increases the risk of cardiovascular disease by 19%. Inflammation from the bacterial infection is believed to be the cause.

---

http://circ-meeting.ahajournals.org/cgi/content/abstract/103/9/1357-b
Oral Surg Oral Med Oral Pathol Oral Radiol Endod. 2003 May;95(5):559-69

Heart

Cranberry juice – the tart that's smart for your heart.

Forget that soda. Drink a glass of cranberry juice.

Here's the science:

A group of volunteers drank cranberry juice three times a day for a month.

Their good cholesterol (HDL) rose by 10%. This correlates to a 40% drop in the risk of heart disease.

They had lower levels of oxidation products in their blood. Cranberries are loaded with antioxidants (including *procyanidins* – red pigments).

http://www.sciencenews.org/articles/20030329/food.asp

Get into the pink of health with purple grape juice.

You don't have to drink wine like a French sailor on shore leave to help your heart. Drinking purple grape juice twice daily improves vascular health.

Here's the science:

Drinking purple grape juice inhibits oxidation of bad cholestrol. Oxidation of LDL in the artery wall triggers plaque formation. The flavonoids (a group of phytochemicals) in purple grape juice are antioxidants that decrease LDL susceptibility to oxidation.

Purple grape juice opens up your arteries. It improves the functioning of the lining of the arteries (endothelium). The endothelium produces nitric oxide (NO), which causes the vessel to dilate and let blood move though more freely.

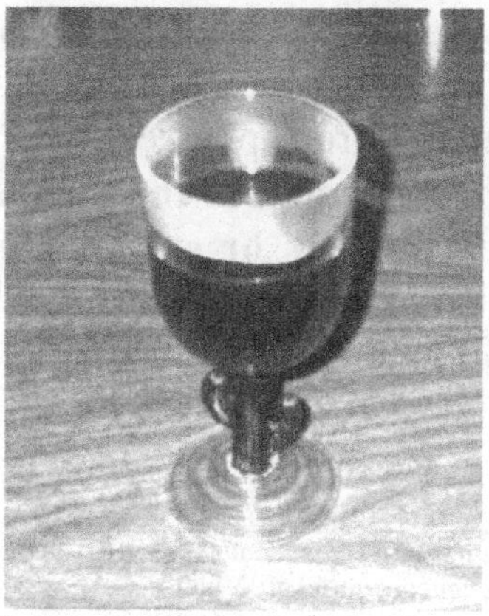

http://circ.ahajournals.org/cgi/content/full/100/10/1050

Heart

Omega-3 – the fat that's phat for your heart.

Add pharmaceutical-grade fish oil supplements to your heart health program. They're a great source of important omega-3 fatty acids.

Here's the science:

Omega-3 fatty acids improve blood lipid profile.

Omega-3 fatty acids have an anti-inflammatory effect.

DHA, one of the omega-3 fatty acids, helps to dilate blood vessels. This contributes to the ability of fish oil to lower blood pressure.

Omega-3 fatty acids keep white blood cells from sticking to the lining of the arteries (endothelium). In vascular disease, white blood cells stick to and enter the artery wall. Inside the artery wall, they gobble up oxidized LDL and become the bloated foam cells associated with fatty streak lesions. Fish oil forestalls the white blood cells' entry.

Omega-3 fatty acids block vascular smooth muscle cell proliferation. The proliferation of smooth muscle cells turns the fatty streak into a fibrous plaque.

Omega-3 fatty acids reduce the formation of clots that can trigger a heart attack or stroke. Omega-3 fatty acids inhibit the production of thromboxane, a compound that stimulates clot formation.

http://circ-meeting.ahajournals.org/cgi/content/abstract/103/9/1351
http://circ.ahajournals.org/cgi/content/full/102/11/1264
http://circ.ahajournals.org/cgi/content/abstract/84/4/1725
http://atvb.ahajournals.org/cgi/content/full/15/2/185
http://circ.ahajournals.org/cgi/content/abstract/108/2/155
http://circ.ahajournals.org/cgi/content/full/102/22/2677
http://atvb.ahajournals.org/cgi/content/full/19/10/2316
Am J Clin Nutr. 1990 Jul; 52(1): 1-28.
http://www.jstage.jst.go.jp/article/jphs/92/4/92_308/_article/-char/en
http://www.nutrition.org/cgi/content/full/134/7/1806
Drugs Today (Barc). 2001 Jan;37(1):49-56.

It's simple, B-complex for better heart health.

Eat a balanced diet including lots of dark-green, leafy vegetables (a good source of the B vitamin folate). For insurance, add a B-complex supplement – or multivitamin – to your heart-health program.

Here's the science:

Homocysteine is a toxic, metabolic by-product. Folate, B_6 and B_{12} help vascular health by suppressing homocyteine levels.

Homocysteine irritates the endothelial cells lining the inside of the arteries. These cells release a chemical call for white blood cells. The entry of white blood cells into the walls of the arteries is a key step in *atherogenesis* – hardening of the arteries.

High homocysteine levels are a risk factor for the formation of clots that can cause heart attacks or strokes.

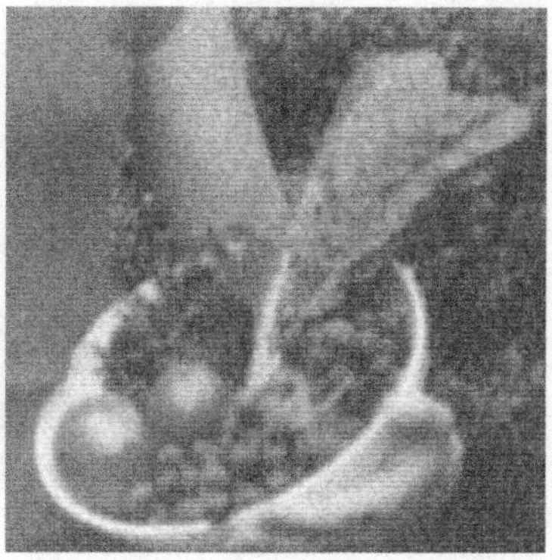

http://circ.ahajournals.org/cgi/content/full/97/5/437
http://circ.ahajournals.org/cgi/content/full/103/22/2717
http://atvb.ahajournals.org/cgi/content/full/22/11/1936
http://atvb.ahajournals.org/cgi/content/abstract/13/9/1327
http://circ-meeting.ahajournals.org/cgi/content/abstract/103/9/1347-e

Heart

D-ribose gets an A+

Do you suffer from chronic coronary heart disease? Ask your doctor about D-ribose supplementation.

Here's the science:

D-ribose supplementation improves the quality of life of patients with chronic coronary heart disease. Three weeks of D-ribose supplementation supports the heart function of patients as measured by echocardiography, a quality of life questionnaire, and cycle ergometer testing.

If you suffer from ischemia, your heart has trouble making the energy molecule ATP. D-ribose supplementation helps ischemia patients' hearts make more ATP.

D-ribose

http://www.ncbi.nlm.nih.gov/entrez/query.fcgi?cmd=Retrieve&db=pubmed&dopt=Abstract&list_uids=14607200

Metabolism and Diabetes

Sprinkle some on.

Do you have – or are at risk for – type 2 diabetes? Sprinkle a teaspoon of ground cinnamon on your oatmeal. (You might also like to try chopped nuts and fresh or dried fruit such as diced apples or dried cranberries.)

Here's the science:

Insulin is a hormone that tells cells to take up glucose from the blood after a meal. Type 2 diabetes is a condition where the cells have a weak response to insulin. Thus they don't take up as much glucose as they should, causing blood glucose to rise.

Phytochemicals in cinnamon potentiate the action of insulin. The cinnamon affects the on/off switches on the cells' insulin receptors, which monitor insulin levels and tell the cell to respond accordingly.

Cinnamon

Biol Trace Elem Res. 1990 Mar;24(3):183-8.
J Agric Food Chem. 2004 Jan 14;52(1):65-70.
http://care.diabetesjournals.org/cgi/content/abstract/26/12/3215
http://content.karger.com/ProdukteDB/produkte.asp?Aktion=ShowAbstract&ProduktNr=224036&Ausgabe=225963&ArtikelNr=23270
J Agric Food Chem. 2000 Mar;48(3):849-52.

Don't be a dumbbell – lift one.

For a better metabolism, do progressive weight training with either free weights or machines.

What do you mean by progressive?

As you get stronger, lift more weight. Don't allow it to become easy.

Here's the science:

Exercising skeletal muscle is the body's largest sink for disposing of excess glucose. Each bout of weight training helps bring glucose levels under control.

A consistent weight-training program can make skeletal muscle a better sink for glucose disposal. Weight training increases the muscle cells' levels of a membrane protein (GLUT-4) that acts like a turnstile, allowing glucose to enter the muscle cell. Exercised muscle cells also make more of the enzymes that process glucose.

Weight training is good for almost everyone. If you have bad knees, you can't jog – but you can sit at a resistance machine and do chest presses. Many elderly individuals with complex medical conditions, such as mobility impairment, tolerate weight training better than aerobic training.

Remember: smart bells lift dumbbells

---

http://care.diabetesjournals.org/cgi/content/full/26/5/1580
Am J Physiol. 1993 Jun;264(6 Pt 1):E896-901.
FEBS Lett. 1990 Jul 30;268(1):13-6.

Metabolism and Diabetes

Don't be cat food.

During Paleolithic times, stress meant you had to run very fast or fight very fiercely so as not to become saber-tooth cat food. You needed a lot of glucose to fuel your muscles. Thus stress triggers hormonal reactions that raise blood glucose levels.

Today, stress might mean catty coworkers at your sedentary job. If you have high blood glucose from diabetes, stress could aggravate it.

Stressed out?

Exercise. Go for a walk or run.

Loose yourself in a hobby. Take you mind off your worries. Discover your talents. Combine this with the above suggestion and get involved in a sport.

Take fish oil supplements.

Here's the science:

Exercise is an especially good way to handle stress because it burns off excess blood glucose and improves metabolism while reducing your stress levels.

The omega-3 fatty acids in fish oil moderate the stress response. The omega-3 fatty acid DHA is a major building block of the brain and deficiency of it affects brain function.

---

http://www.eurekalert.org/pub_releases/2002-08/apa-psm081302.php
http://care.diabetesjournals.org/cgi/content/full/25/1/30
http://www.eurekalert.org/pub_releases/1997-04/Uola-SBOE-030497.php
Diabetes Metab. 2003 Jun;29(3):289-95.

Metabolism and Diabetes

Take a hike.

Taking long (more than 30 minutes), brisk, daily walks can help prevent type 2 diabetes. Push yourself to walk briskly enough to be breathing heavier but not so fast that you can't talk.

Here's the science:

Exercise burns glucose, thus lowering your blood glucose level with each bout of exercise.

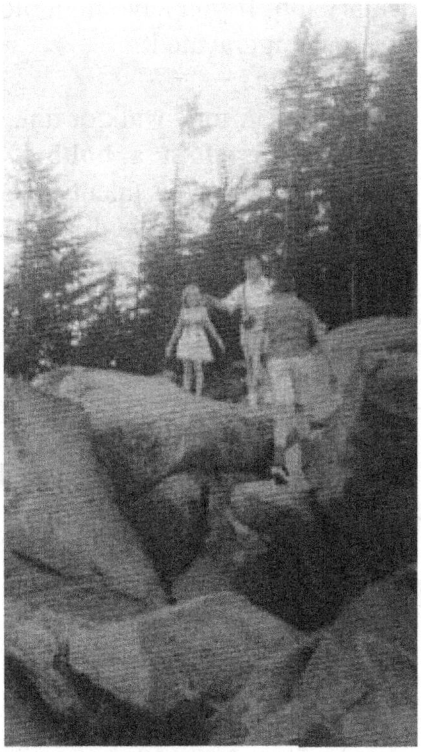

Frequent exercise stimulates your muscle cells to make more GLUT-4. GLUT-4 acts like a turnstile, allowing glucose to leave the blood and enter the muscle cells.

Exercised muscle cells make more of the enzymes that process glucose. Muscle cells store and utilize glucose in multi-step processes. Enzymes catalyze – assist in – the reactions.

---

http://www.eurekalert.org/pub_releases/2002-06/uopm-daw061302.php
http://www.eurekalert.org/pub_releases/2003-09/uopm-ecr092403.php
http://www.eurekalert.org/pub_releases/2003-08/mc-mcs081503.php
FEBS Lett. 1990 Jul 30;268(1):13-6.
JAMA. 1999 Oct 20;282(15):1433-9.

Metabolism and Diabetes

Mg – magnificent.

Magnesium normalizes blood glucose levels. In order to get more magnesium in your diet, eat nuts, whole grains, and dark green, leafy vegetables. If you have or are at risk for type 2 diabetes, take a magnesium supplement.

Here's the science:

Magnesium aids glucose metabolism and insulin action. It's a cofactor for several enzymes involved in carbohydrate metabolism. Magnesium is also critical for the action of insulin in muscle cells.

People whose diets are low in magnesium have an increased risk of type 2 diabetes. Animals on a low magnesium diet get type 2 diabetes, too.

Magnesium supplementation prevents type 2 diabetes in rats on a high sugar diet. High carbohydrate foods require more magnesium to metabolize; however, magnesium is processed out of sugar and refined grains.

Magnesium supplementation is recommended for individuals with type 2 diabetes. Patients see improved insulin-mediated glucose uptake with magnesium supplementation.

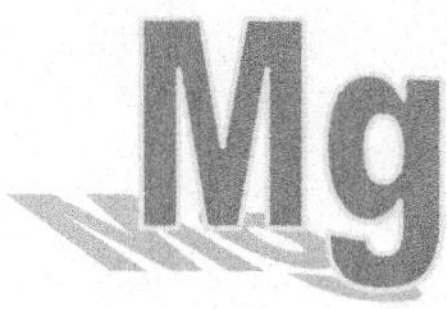

---

http://www.sciencedirect.com/science?_ob=ArticleURL&_udi=B6T0Y-3S0W7Y9-J&_coverDate=03%2F31%2F1997&_alid=184796617&_rdoc=1&_fmt=&_orig=search&_qd=1&_cdi=4875&_sort=d&view=c&_acct=C000050221&_version=1&_urlVersion=0&_userid=10&md5=9174b459c12b4545dbb72571d356814e

Mol Aspects Med. 2003 Feb-Jun;24(1-3):39-52.

http://care.diabetesjournals.org/cgi/content/full/27/1/134

http://care.diabetesjournals.org/cgi/content/full/27/1/59

http://hyper.ahajournals.org/cgi/content/abstract/23/6/1036

Get some Zzzzzzzzzzs.

Science has proven the folk wisdom that it pays to get a good night's sleep.

Here's the science:

Wrestling with a difficult problem?

A good night's sleep might help you find a solution. In an article published in Nature, researchers presented the subjects with a problem and tested them on it. They were retested on it eight hours later. Compared with subjects who'd been awake during the eight-hour break, subjects who'd slept during that time did significantly better on the retest. The researchers concluded that sleep restructures new memory representations, facilitating insight.

So get your Zzzzzzzzzzzs.

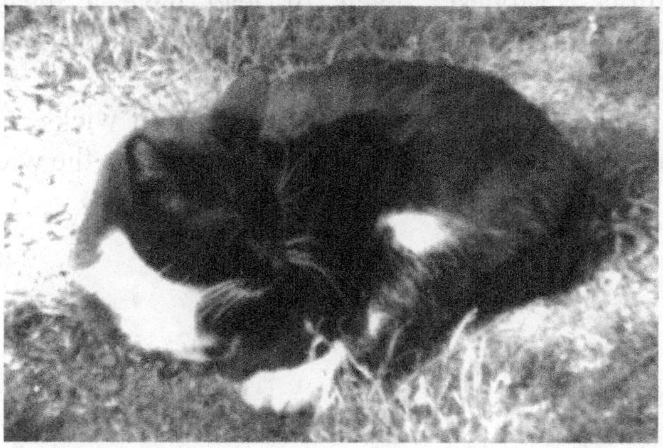

Shhhhh. I'm working on the unified field theory.

Nature. 2004 Jan 22; 427(6972): 352-5
http://www.sciencenews.org/20020907/bob9.asp

Do your candles have wicked wicks?

When shopping for candles, check the tip of the wicks. If the wick has a dark, metallic center, don't purchase the candle!

Here's the science:

Wicks with lead or lead-containing-metal-alloy cores are often used in candles to provide a slower burn rate. However, upon burning, the lead becomes volatilized. In an enclosed room, a single candle can cause the concentration of lead in the air to reach levels up to several times greater than the EPA limit. Multiple candles result in even higher levels. Repeated exposure may induce clinical lead poisoning. The neuropsychological effects of lead poisoning include irritability, psychiatric symptoms, and learning disabilities. "Modest" levels of lead have a measurable psychological affect in adults and cause learning impairment in children.

Fortunately, not all candles have wicked wicks. Candles can be fun and romantic – as long as you check the wick.

Sci Total Environ 2002 Sep 16;296(1-3):159-74
Sci Total Environ 2000 Apr 24;250(1-3):37-41
Sci Total Environ 1999 Dec 15;243-244:53-65
J Occup Environ Med. 2003 Nov;45(11):1144-51.
http://www.eurekalert.org/pub_releases/2003-04/nioe-vll041503.php

A berry smart dessert.

For dessert, have a bowl of blueberries instead of cake.

Here's the science:

Research on elderly rodents has shown that blueberries have the power to reverse age-related neurodegenerative disease. Blueberry supplementation gave the elderly rodents better balance and coordination. They had superior working memory. Their neurochemistry was better than the control group.

In a separate set of experiments, mice genetically predisposed toward Alzheimer's disease were feed blueberry supplementation from a youthful age. The blueberry-munching rodents resisted developing Alzheimer's later on.

What gives blueberries these super powers? It's due to their blend of phytonutrients called flavonoids – particularly anthocyanins.

Flavonoids are antioxidants. They quench free radicals – highly reactive by-products of metabolism. Antioxidants keep free radicals from damaging the various components of the cell.

Favonoids enhance cell membrane fluidity. The biophysical properties of membranes influence the activity of proteins in the membrane. If the membrane is too rigid, some membrane proteins don't work as well. Would you want to do water aerobics in a pool filled with molasses?

Flavonoids have anti-inflammatory activity. Inflammation contributes to Alzheimer's disease and strokes.

Nutr Neurosci 2003 Jun; 6(3): 153-62
http://www.jneurosci.org/cgi/content/full/19/18/8114
Ann N Y Acad Sci 2002 Apr; 959: 128-32
J Med Food. 2001 Spring; 4(1): 49-51
Adv Exp Med Biol. 1996; 408: 179-83.

Patriot's Parfait

Sliced strawberries
Blue berries
Vanilla yogurt

Place a layer of vanilla yogurt in parfait glasses. Add a layer of blue berries. Add another layer of vanilla yogurt. Add a layer of sliced strawberries. Top off with vanilla yogurt. Serve.

Freedom Fruit Cups

1 pint strawberries
1 pint blueberries
2 apples

Slice strawberries. Cut the apples into bite-sized chunks. Toss. Portion into fruit cups. Serve.

Yield: serves six.

Read – learn something new and grow a better brain.

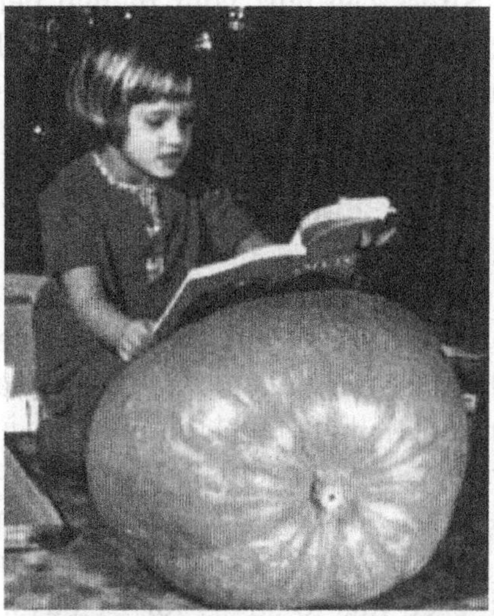

Interested in nature? Explore the ocean depths, the wild apple forests of Kazakhstan, and more through books. Bored? History books detailing a dramatic event can transport you to a different time and place. Not only will you gain new insights on the topic you read about, you will build a more powerful brain.

Here's the science:

Rodents housed in enriched environments show increased *neurogenesis* – growing new brain cells, enhanced learning ability, and decreased age-dependent degeneration of the brain.

However, the toys that rats find cognitively stimulating might not excite you. And while spending the rest of your life on a world cruise probably isn't within your budget, you can transport your *mind* to far-off places, even time-travel, through books. Informal continuing education – reading – can enrich your mental environment and build your brain.

Ann Neurol. 2002 Aug; 52(2): 135-43.
J Neurobiol. 1999 Jun 15; 39(4): 569-78.
http://www.applejournal.com/bk003.htm

Mind

Beat stress before it beats you.

Stress can hurt your mental performance. To beat stress, exercise and take fish oil, vitamin B complex, and vitamin C supplements.

Here's the science:

Stress initiates a chain reaction starting in the pre-frontal cortex of the brain. Along the way, the acute stress hormones epinephrine and norepinephrine are released. These fight or flight hormones give you a quick jolt of alarm. Chronic stress results in the increased release of cortisol. A sustained high level of cortisol is toxic to the part of the brain (the hippocampus) involved in memory and emotional stability – damage to the hippocampus leads to depression.

Stress hurts the brains of mice and men. Scientists exposed rats to stress for 21 days. They found that the rats' hippocampal expression of a molecule that lets neurons reach out and touch one another was decreased. Other studies reveal that prolonged exposure to cortisol causes hippocampal neurons to shrivel and die. In humans, years of severe stress can cause the hippocampus to shrink up to 26 percent.

The good news is that exercise can help. The stress-reactive brain circuits in the pre-frontal cortex of rats that regularly exercised responded less to stress.

Neuro Plast. 2002; 9(3): 147-59.
Bipolar Disord.2002 Apr; 4(2):117-28.
http://www.sciencenews.org/sn_arc99/9_4_99/note5ref.htm
http://www.eurekalert.org/pub_releases/1999-10/UoCa-Csse-241099.php
http://www.eurekalert.org/pub_releases/1999-10/DUMC-DsEm-231099.php
http://www.eurekalert.org/pub_releases/1999-06/WUSo-Hshl-150699.php
http://www.eurekalert.org/pub_releases/1996-08/SU-NSOH-150896.php
New Scientist. 2004;182(2445):42-45.
http://www.e2med.com/index.cfm?fuseaction=viewArtDossier&DartIdx=151325&DIssIdx=8801&DChapIdx=66135

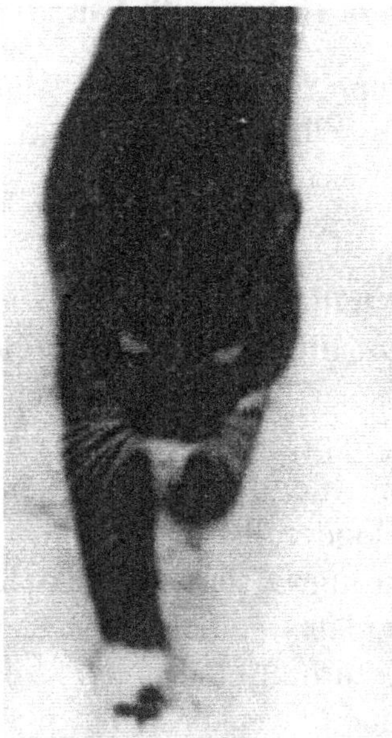

Let's see, stress can cause osteoporosis, cancer, hardening of the arteries, high blood sugar, poor memory, and depression. But exercise can help. Well then, let's play!

Get into the swim of things with fish oil supplements.

Take fish oil supplements to feed your brain. Fish oil is used to treat stress, depression, autism, Alzheimer's, and Parkinson's.

Here's the science:

Fish oil is high in the omega-3 fatty acids EPA and DHA.

EPA is an anti-inflammatory nutrient. Inflammation contributes to vascular disease, which can lead to a stroke. Inflamed arteries express molecules on their inner wall, which cause white blood cells to enter the arterial wall. There the white blood cells gobble up oxidized LDL – bad cholesterol – causing a fatty streak lesion to develop. Inflammation stimulates smooth muscle cells in the artery wall to multiply, turning the fatty streak into a fibrous plaque. Inflammation weakens the plaque. Debris from disruption of the plaque can block smaller vessels downstream and cause a stroke.

Inflammation also contributes to Alzheimer's disease.

DHA is a vital component of the nerve cell membrane. Nerve cells need to have enough of it to function properly. Research on rats has determined that a deficiency of DHA leads to a decreased learning ability. DHA protects the synapses – connections between brain cells – of mice that were genetically designed to develop Alzheimer's disease.

---

http://www.thorne.com/altmedrev/.fulltext/8/4/410.pdf
J Lipid Res. 2003 Dec; 44(12): 2221-33. Epub 2003 Sep 16
Altern Med Rev. 2003 Nov; 8(4): 410-25
Arch Neurol. 2003 Jul;60(7):940-6.
Can J Psychiatry. 2003 Apr; 48(3): 195-203.
Behav Neurosci. 2002 Dec; 116(6): 1022-31.
Prostaglandins Leukot Essent Fatty Acids. 2001 Jul;65(1):1-7.
Int J Dev Neurosci. 2000 Jul-Aug; 18(4-5): 383-99.
http://www.eurekalert.org/pub_releases/2004-09/uoc--ddp082604.php
http://www.e2med.com/index.cfm?fuseaction=viewArtDossier&DartIdx=151325&DIssIdx=8801&DChapIdx=66135

Move your muscles, build your brain.

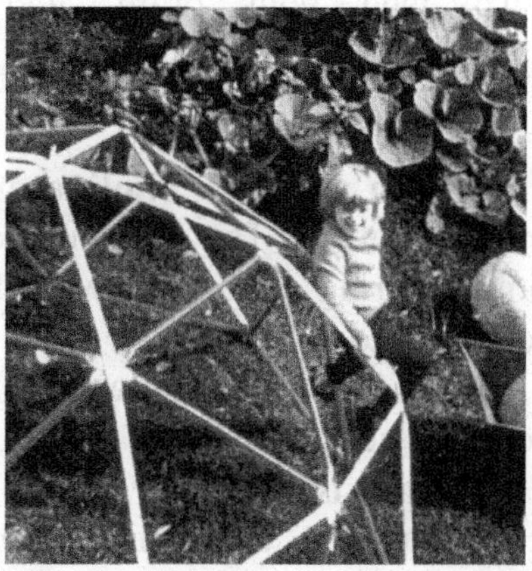

No matter what your age, physical activity is important for superior mental performance.

Here's the science: **Exercise helps you grow new brain cells** (neurogenesis) by maintaining healthy levels of BDNF and other growth factors in the brain. And yes, even adults can grow new neurons.

Exercise keeps stress from burning out your brain. Brain damage due to chronic stress is one pathway to depression.

Chronic stress results in unhealthy, high levels of the hormone cortisol, which damage a region of the brain called the hippocampus. Damage to this area of the brain from stress is a major pathway to depression.

Exercise training helps to regulate cortisol levels. In addition, since exercise stimulates neurogenesis, it counteracts the damage caused by stress.

Walking can help prevent dementia. A recent study found that senior women who engage in regular exercise perform better on cognitive tests.

Trends Neurosci. 2002 Jun;25(6):295-301.
Neuroscience. 2004;124(4):985-92.
http://www.nature.com/cgi-taf/DynaPage.taf?file=/neuro/journal/v2/n3/abs/nn0399_266.html
Chin J Physiol. 2001 Mar 31;44(1):13-8.
New Scientist.2004;182(24450):42-45.
http://www.eurekalert.org/pub_releases/2004-09/jaaj-pai091604.php

Let's get lecithin.

To feed your brain, add lecithin to your daily supplements.

Here's the science:

Lecithin contains choline, an important nutrient for brain function. The offspring of rats given supplemental choline during pregnancy were found to have an increased memory size.

Choline is part of the membrane that surrounds cells, including nerve cells.

Choline is the percusor to the neurotransmitter acetylcholine – a chemical used to send signals between certain nerve cells. Acetylcholine is used by the neurons in the hippocampus – a part of the brain involved in memory formation.

Lecithin

http://www.sciencenews.org/articles/20011103/bob13.asp

Mind

Purple power for seniors.

Replace that soda with purple grape juice. The switch will help keep you mentally young.

Here's the science:

Elderly rats that chugged Concord (purple) grape juice performed better on memory and neuro-motor skills tests. That's because it's not just blueberries that have neuroprotective phytochemicals, purple grape juice is rich in some too.

Quercetin, an important nutrient for brain health, works through multiple mechanisms.

Quercetin, an antioxidant, protects the brain from free radicals.

Quercetin decreases the activity of COX-2. COX-2 activity stimulates plaque formation in Alzheimer's disease.

Quercetin is also a vasodilator. It aids blood flow to the brain.

Resveratrol, another antioxidant, protects neuronal *mitochondria* – the powerhouses of the cell – during a stroke.

Kaempferol is found in purple grape juice. But it's also one of the factors responsible for ginkgo biloba's neuroprotective action.

---

http://www.eurekalert.org/pub_releases/2003-12/jai-cgj121803.php
http://www.scielo.br/scielo.php?script=sci_arttext&pid=S0100-879X2003001200002&lng=en&nrm=iso
http://www.sciencedirect.com/science?_ob=ArticleURL&_udi=B6T38-4BBH64H-2&_coverDate=03%2F01%2F2004&_alid=175774068&_rdoc=1&_fmt=&_orig=search&_qd=1&_cdi=4940&_sort=d&view=c&_acct=C000050221&_version=1&_urlVersion=0&_userid=10&md5=1f2c688dc9cff73f664a4afb137d214d
http://www.thieme-connect.com/DOI/DOI?10.1055/s-2003-45144
http://www3.interscience.wiley.com/cgi-bin/abstract/93520069/ABSTRACT
Drugs Exp Clin Res. 2003;29(5-6):227-33.
J Pharm Pharmacol. 2000 Apr;52(4):451-9.
Gene Expr. 2002;10(5-6):271-8.
Curr Drug Targets. 2003 Aug;4(6):461-8.

Pain – Lower Back

Get back into action.

Back pain? Try water exercise or Tai Chi.

Water supports you while giving you light resistance. Aquatic exercise – water aerobics – classes are offered at many fitness centers and YMCAs/YWCAs.

Tai Chi was originally developed as a martial art. It later evolved to focus on health. Tai Chi limbers the body while gently toning muscles.

Here's the science:

Major causes of low back pain are poor physical conditioning of the torso, stiffness in the hamstrings, excess weight, and stress.

Water exercise and Tai Chi are gentle exercises that condition the torso and increase hamstring flexibility. They're manageable for most beginners. Conditioning your torso and stretching your hamstrings can often alleviate back pain.

Moderate to vigorous physical activity is an important part of a weight loss program. However, low back pain precludes participation in many forms of exercise. Water exercise and Tai Chi are gentle enough for most people. For weight loss you may wish to add other exercises – such as brisk walking or running when you are ready.

Stress can cause back injury. When you're under negative psychological stress, you tense your muscles differently. This can cause you to lift heavy objects incorrectly, which places more stress on your spine and can lead to injury. Moderate exercise, such as water aerobics, decreases stress hormone levels.

---

http://orthoinfo.aaos.org/brochure/thr_report.cfm?Thread_ID=10&topcategory=Spine
Pain. 2004 Jan;107(1-2):176-90.
http://www.jstage.jst.go.jp/article/jpa/19/4/19_175/_article/-char/en
http://www.eurekalert.org/pub_releases/2000-11/OSU-Jsml-3011100.php
Kurume Med J. 1999;46(2):91-6.

Pain – PAD

B pain-free.

Peripheral arterial disease (PAD) produces pain in the legs, which makes walking difficult. It's caused by poor circulation from hardening of the arteries.

Do you want to keep some spring in your step as you get older? Eat plenty of dark-green, leafy vegetables (a good source of the B vitamin folate) and take a B-complex supplement or multivitamin for insurance.

Here's the science:

Folate helps keep your arteries healthy. High plasma homocysteine damages the inner surface of blood vessels and can lead to cardiovascular problems including. PAD. Vitamin B-complex, especially folate, helps reduce homocysteine levels. A Harvard study found that men who had higher intakes of folate had a 33% lower risk of developing PAD.

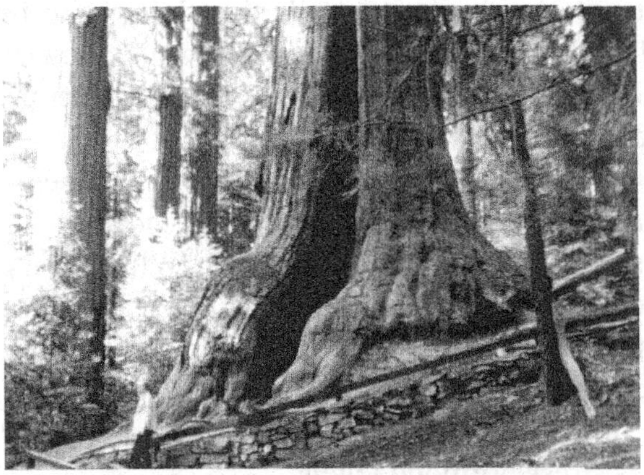

Do you want to take walks to see the foliage when you get older? Then eat some dark-green, leafy vegetables and take folate supplements now.

---

http://www.nutrition.org/cgi/content/full/133/9/2863

Pain and Inflammation

Oil change.

Use canola oil instead of vegetable oil in your cooking.

While fish oil contains the important omega-3 fatty acids EPA and DHA, flaxseed and canola oils contain another omega-3 fatty acid, ALA.

Humans evolved eating a Paleolithic diet which contained an even balance of omega-6 to omega-3 fatty acids. Over the past century, this ratio has been drastically altered by increased consumption of omega-6 fatty acids from corn oil, sunflower seed oil, safflower seed oil, cottonseed oil, and soybean oil. Our diet is now 20:1 omega-6 to omega-3 fatty acids.

How can you balance your omegas? In addition to taking fish oil supplements, replace that bottle of vegetable oil in your pantry with canola oil. Canola oil has a lower omega-6 to omega-3 ratio than many other cooking oils. Flaxseed oil isn't good for cooking (it smokes upon heating) but flaxseed meal can add a nutty flavor to your baking.

Here's the science:

ALA → EPA + DHA. The body has a limited ability to convert the short-chain fatty acid ALA into the important long-chain fatty acids EPA and DHA. However, consumption of large amounts of the omega-6 fatty acid LA blocks this reaction.

Omega-6 fatty acids are the building blocks for eicosanoids that cause inflammation.

---

http://www.ajcn.org/cgi/content/full/70/3/560S

Pain

Inflamed? Go fishin'

Does inflammation have you feeling down? Try fish oil supplements – a rich source of the omega-3 fatty acids including EPA.

Here's the science:

EPA inhibits the production of molecules that cause pain and inflammation.

EPA suppresses the production of omega-6-derived eicosanoids by COX-2. These eicosanoids cause pain and inflammation.

EPA inhibits the production of cytokines, which cause inflammation.

Omega-3 fatty acids act on the nervous system. This may contribute to their ability to reduce feelings of pain.

---

http://www.scielo.br/scielo.php?script=sci_arttext&pid=S0100-879X2003000400004&tlng=es&lng=en&nrm=iso
http://www.ncbi.nlm.nih.gov/entrez/query.fcgi?cmd=Retrieve&db=pubmed&dopt=Abstract&list_uids=12591006
http://www.jacn.org/cgi/content/abstract/21/6/495
http://www.ncbi.nlm.nih.gov/entrez/query.fcgi?cmd=Retrieve&db=pubmed&dopt=Abstract&list_uids=15294488

Pain

When you're feeling in the pits…

Achy joints or sore muscles? Tart cherry extract reduces inflammatory pain in rats.

But do you have to eat *tart* cherries? Sweet cherries have some of the active compounds found in tart cherries so sweet cherries would be of some benefit too.

Cherries out of season? Dried cherries are available at some grocery and Walmart stores. Tart cherry extract capsules are available at health food stores.

Here's the science:

Cherry red is soothing. Anthocyanins – red phytochemicals found in cherries – reduce inflammation by inhibiting COX enzymes, the targets of anti- inflammatory drugs such as aspirin.

Cherry red neutralizes free radicals generated by inflammation. Anthocyanins are potent antioxidants.

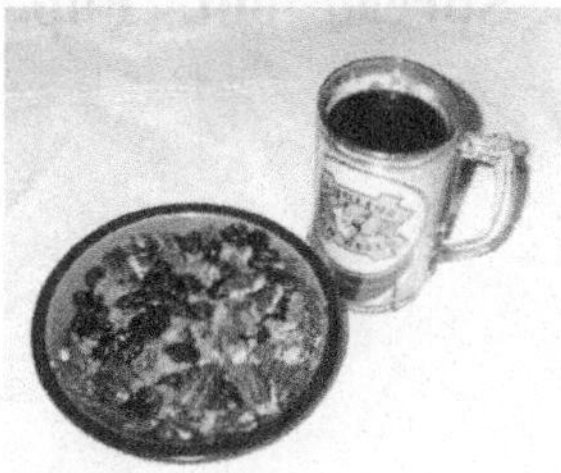

For a super-healthy, game-time snack, try mixing dried cherries, chopped dates, and salt-free nuts.

Behav Brain Res. 2004 Aug 12; 153(1):181-8
http://www.eurekalert.org/pub_releases/1999-01/ACS-NPAS-280199.php
http://www.ncbi.nlm.nih.gov/entrez/query.fcgi?cmd=Retrieve&db=pubmed&dopt=Abstract&list_uids=14759143
http://www.ncbi.nlm.nih.gov/entrez/query.fcgi?cmd=Retrieve&db=pubmed&dopt=Abstract&list_uids=11600045

Very Cherry Hotcakes
1 cup whole wheat flour
½ cup Splenda
2 teaspoon baking powder
½ teaspoon salt
1¼ cups soy milk
¼ cup canola oil
1 cage-free egg
2 cups dried cherries
½ cup cranberry juice

Place 2 cups of dried cherries in a zipper-type plastic bag. Add cranberry juice. Place in refrigerator overnight so the cherries will soften.

Mix dry ingredients. Add wet other ingredients. Mix. Add cherries. Mix. Pour ½ cup at a time onto a preheated oiled frying pan. Spread out. Flip. Serve. Top with applesauce.

Yield: 6 hotcakes.

Fight pain with phytochemicals.

Do you have joint pain? Old injuries acting up? Put more fruits and veggies in your diet.

A diet deficient in fruits and vegetables can predispose the body to inflammation. However, few people eat the recommended eight or more servings per day. This may be one reason why inflammatory conditions are so common.

What's a serving? A serving is one cup of lettuce or a half cup of fruit or vegetable. Choose mostly brightly colored produce such as blueberries or carrots. Those bright colors are phytochemicals.

Here's the science:

Elderly who eat more fruit and vegetables have less inflammation. A diet rich in fruits and vegetables is associated with lower levels of C-reactive protein and plasma total homocysteine – markers of inflammation.

Supplementing elderly rats' diets with apples decreases their levels of proinflammatory cytokines. Apple skins are rich in antioxidant phytochemicals, which help to decrease inflammation.

Certain fruit phytochemicals reduce COX-2 activity. COX-2 makes chemicals (eicosanoids) that cause inflammation.

fight-o-chemicals

---

http://www.ncbi.nlm.nih.gov/entrez/query.fcgi?cmd=Retrieve&db=pubmed&dopt=Abstract&list_uids=11986578
http://www.ncbi.nlm.nih.gov/entrez/query.fcgi?cmd=Retrieve&db=pubmed&dopt=Abstract&list_uids=15051846
http://www.jneurosci.org/cgi/content/full/22/14/6114
Mutat Res. 2004 Jul 13;551(1-2):245-54.

Here's an easy way you can put some fight-o-chemicals in your diet:

<u>Honey Do Dinner</u>

Honey dew melon
2 cups sliced strawberries
2 cups blueberries
1 cup chopped pecans

Cut melon in half and deseed. Slice strawberries. (No you don't have to chop the pecans – you can find chopped pecans in the baking aisle of the grocery store.)Toss sliced strawberries, blueberries, and chopped pecans in a bowl. Scoop fruit salad into melon halves. Serve.

Yield: dinner for two.

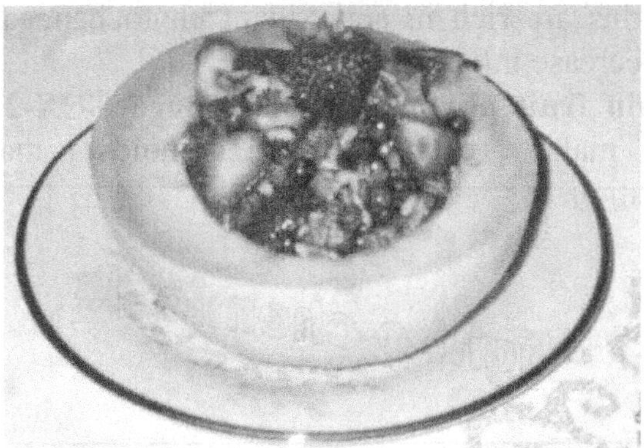

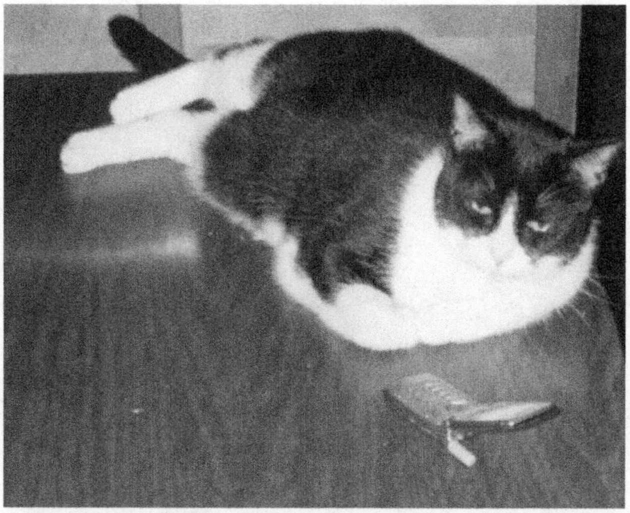

Let's see, COX-2 makes bad-bad stuff that causes cancer, heart disease, Alzheimer's, and pain. But you can control COX-2 with aspirin, fight-o-chemicals, and fishy oil. I'm calling for a take-out order of sushi – that's fishy.

Weight Control

Get an hourglass figure – exercise an hour a day.

Our bodies evolved during the Stone Age when physical activity was a fact of life. That's no longer the case. We don't have to hunt down our dinner with spears. We don't have to climb trees to get apples. We don't have to walk miles to find blueberry bushes. The result is an epidemic of obesity. These days, we have to purposefully put physical activity back into our lives.

Start out at 30 minutes a day of exercise and work your way up to an hour a day. Try a variety of activities to prevent boredom – walking, resistance training, kickboxing, dancing, swimming, water aerobics, etc. – variety is the spice of life.

Here's the science:

Modern life has a darker side. Modern technology has nearly eliminated physical activity from our lives. Even childhood play is becoming sedentary with computer games. As a result, obesity rates are climbing. Those extra pounds increase the risk of type 2 diabetes, heart disease, and cancer. "Today's kids may be the first generation in history whose life expectancy is projected to be less than that of their parents," stated Yale public-health expert, Dr. David Katz.

---

http://www.eurekalert.org/pub_releases/2003-09/uopm-prf090803.php
http://www.ajcn.org/cgi/content/abstract/79/5/913S
http://www.foxnews.com/story/0,2933,130345,00.html
Med Clin North Am. 2000 Mar;84(2):419-40.
http://www.time.com/time/subscriber/covers/1101040607/article/how_we_grew_so_big_diet01a.html

Weight Control

White – out.

Choose whole-grain products instead of white bread.

Here's the science:

A Harvard study found that the more refined grains women ate, the heavier they were. Women who ate high-fiber, whole-grain products tended to be leaner.

Am J Clin Nutr. 2003 Nov;78(5):920-7.

Weight Control

Turn off the blubber tube.

Turn off the tube, go outside, and play.

Need to keep up with favorite programs? Ride an exercise bike or walk on a treadmill while watching them.

Here's the science:

Teens who watch less TV weigh less. Teens are 40% less likely to be overweight if they watch one hour or less of TV per day than if they watch it four or more hours a day.

Women who watch more TV are heavier. A Harvard study found that television watching increased women's risk of obesity.

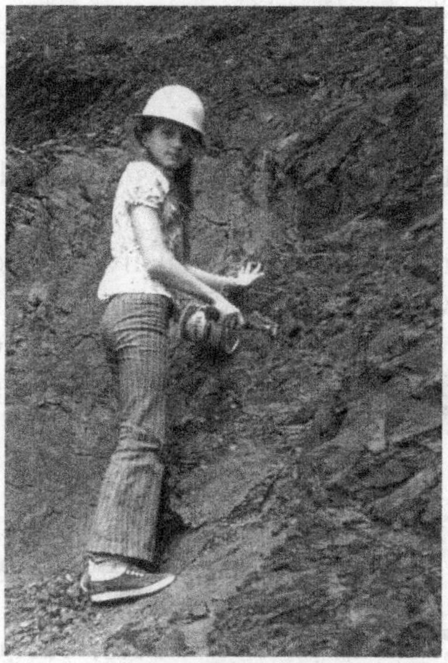

Instead of spending the weekend watching the tube, go rock hounding and find some gems.

Obes Res. 2002 May;10(5):379-85.
JAMA. 2003 Apr 9;289(14):1785-91.

A vigorous hobby or two, makes for a slimmer you.

Martial Arts. Tae Kwon Do is great for toning your legs. Former wrestlers often gravitate toward Judo, a Japanese grappling art. People of all ages get a good workout with Tai Chi.

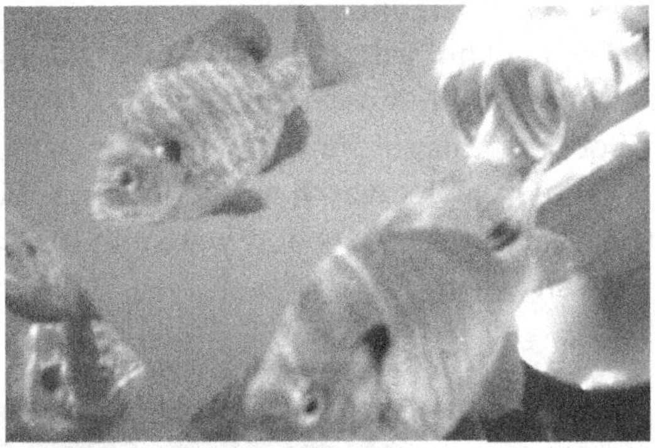

Snorkeling. Even if you don't live by a tropical beach, there may be a great snorkeling spot in your area. Many old rock quarries have been converted to dive resorts. They're stocked with lots of friendly fish.

Hiking. Get a good pair of shoes and explore the parks in your area.

Cross Country Skiing. If you live up north, you might like to try this very vigorous wintertime activity.

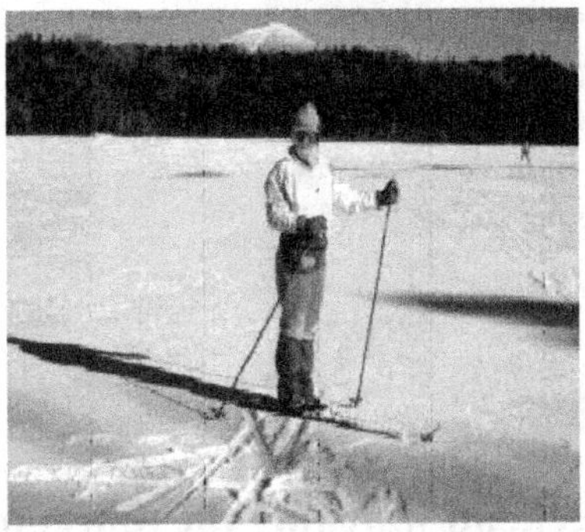

Dance Classes. From ballroom dancing to jazz dancing to folk dancing to belly dancing, there is a style to suit most people.

Also there's canoeing, tennis, golf (no cart), 10K races, racquetball, squash, snow shoeing, ice skating....

Use positive reinforcement.

Even a rat knows it'll run a maze more if it gets a rat treat at the end. After your workout, treat yourself to aromatherapy soap.

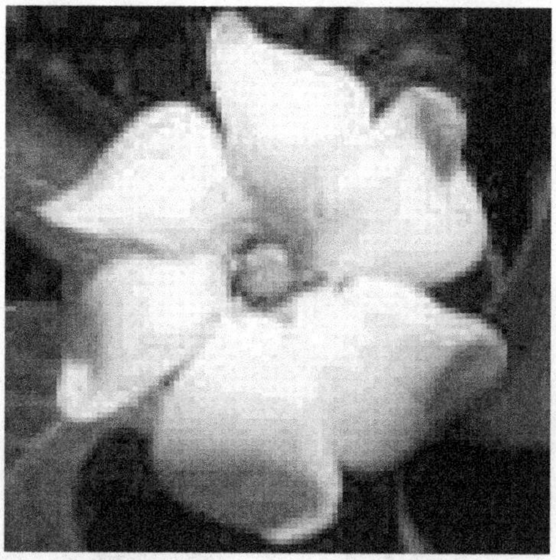

Weight Control

Go for the gold!

Athletic competition is a great motivating factor for vigorous training.

Beyond a certain age? Try masters' division competition.

Bonus: you get to take vacations at competition locations!

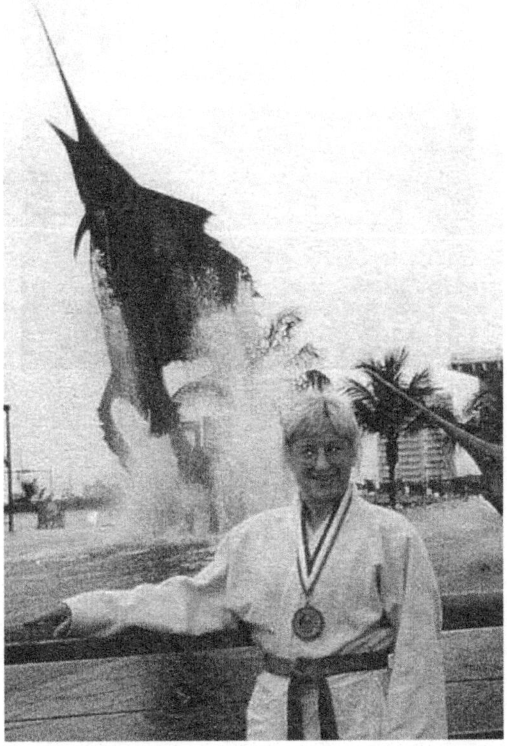

Weight Control

Sleep away the pounds.

Sleep deprivation has numerous detrimental effects on the body. It may even make you obese. So don't drink caffeinated beverages in the evening. And simplify your life so you have time to sleep.

Here's the science:

Chronic sleep deficiency reduces 24-hour leptin concentrations – a hormone that signals satiety. Leptin deficiency makes your body think that you're starving. Reduced leptin concentrations may explain why sleep deprived people tend to snack on junk foods.

So get some beauty (and health) rest.

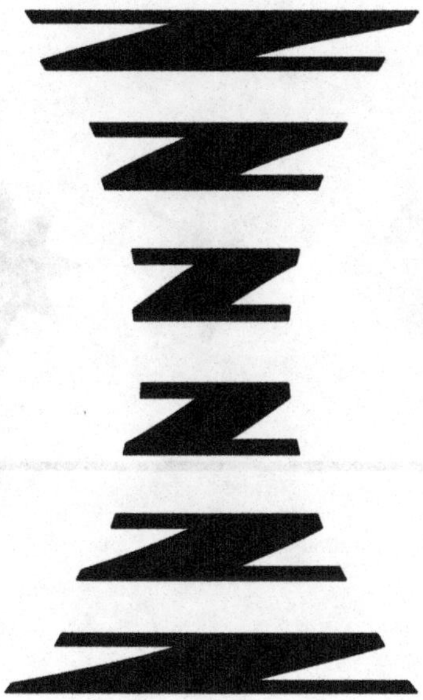

http://www.sciencenews.org/20020907/bob9ref.asp

Give yourself a star.

Track your workouts by drawing stars on a calendar. Use colorful marker pens so you can color code what type of exercise you did. Example: red for brisk walking and blue for resistance training. Draw a star for every 15 minutes of exercise you do. Example: two red stars for a brisk 30 minute walk and one blue star for 15 minutes of resistance training.

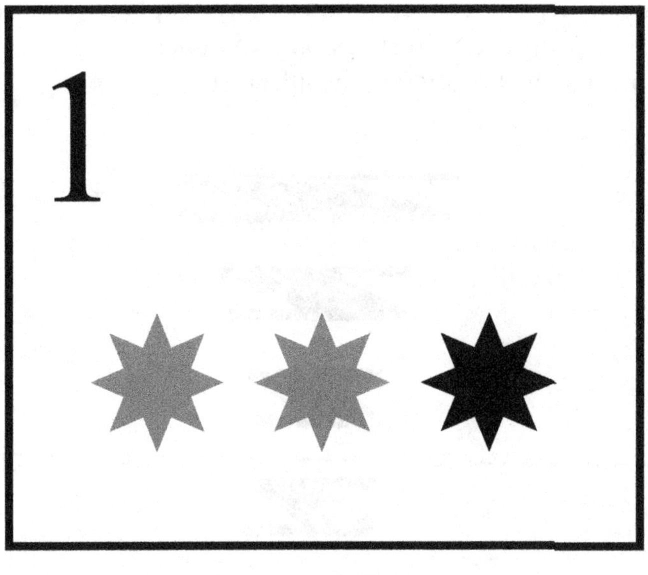

Baby yourself.

Many dieters find success with eating six mini-meals per day. Here's another idea for a mini-meal that doesn't take a lot of time to prepare – a jar of baby-food such as turkey and vegetable dinner. It's fast, convenient – just unscrew the lid – and has balanced nutrition. Baby food is better for you than most energy bars. It tastes good too!

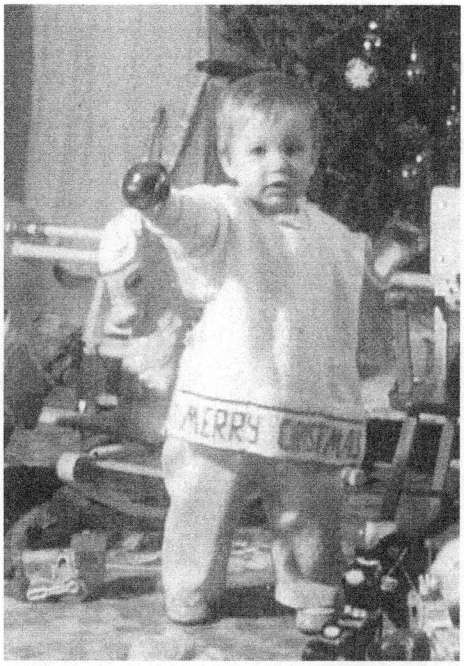

Rediscover the pleasures of your youth.

Weight Control

That's grape!

Add grape seed extract supplements to your diet and exercise program.

Here's the science:

The phytochemicals in grape seed extract decrease fattiness by:

Decreasing hunger.

Altering fat metabolism. It inhibits fat absorption and the accumulation of fat in fatty tissue.

Bonus: Grape seed extract is rich in procyanidins – a class of phytochemicals. This gives it additional health benefits due to its antioxidant activity.

---

http://www.nature.com/cgi-taf/DynaPage.taf?file=/ejcn/journal/v58/n4/abs/1601863a.html
http://www.sciencedirect.com/science?_ob=ArticleURL&_udi=B6TB0-49PX515-C&_coverDate=10%2F31%2F2003&_alid=177273670&_rdoc=1&_fmt=&_orig=search&_qd=1&_cdi=5128&_sort=d&view=c&_acct=C000050221&_version=1&_urlVersion=0&_userid=10&md5=aa6e227eea4c1dda90788a0d0b65d854
Free Radic Res. 2003 May;37(5):573-84.

They'll be green with envy.

Add green tea to your diet and exercise program.

Here's the science:
Green tea contains anti-fattiness phytochemicals:
Catechins – enhance your ability to burn fat by inhibiting the breakdown of norepinephrine. Norepinephrine helps burn fat.
Theanine – an anti-obesity phytochemical.
Caffeine – promotes thermogenesis – burning calories for heat.

Bonus: The phytochemicals in green tea have other health benefits as well.

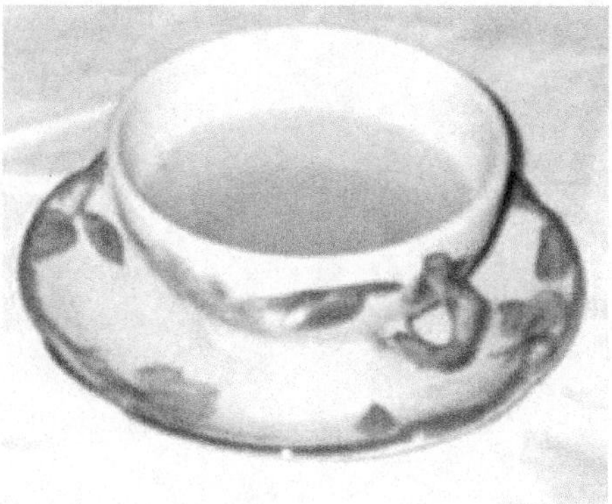

http://www.ajcn.org/cgi/content/full/70/6/1040
In Vivo. 2004 Jan-Feb;18(1):55-62.
http://www.sciencenews.org/articles/20030920/food.asp
http://www.eurekalert.org/pub_releases/2004-05/cmc-aco051704.php

Wound

Spice is nice.

Curcumin, a phytochemical found in the spice turmeric, enhances wound healing. If you don't care for spicy food, you can get curcumin in capsule form.

Here's how curcumin work:

Curcumin is an antioxidant. Wounds experience oxidative stress, which is partially abated through antioxidant supplementation.

Curcumin speed healing of skin by increasing the expression of a growth factor at the wound site. The growth factor binds to the cell surface triggering a series of reactions, which switches on genes involved in healing.

Curcumin helps muscle healing by regulating a transcription factor – a chemical which turns specific genetic switches – so that some of your baby muscle cells (myoblasts) mature and patch up the muscle.

spicy

---

http://www.sciencedirect.com/science?_ob=ArticleURL&_udi=B6TWB-49P48GF-2&_coverDate=05%2F31%2F2004&_alid=177560176&_rdoc=1&_fmt=&_orig=search&_qd=1&_cdi=5558&_sort=d&view=c&_acct=C000050221&_version=1&_urlVersion=0&_userid=10&md5=55a8f7c6ff2c2d9c658ff5f4c44238f1

http://www.blackwell-synergy.com/openurl?genre=article&sid=nlm:pubmed&issn=1067-1927&date=1998&volume=6&issue=2&spage=167

http://www.blackwell-synergy.com/openurl?genre=article&sid=nlm:pubmed&issn=1067-1927&date=1999&volume=7&issue=5&spage=362

http://www.jtrauma.com/pt/re/jtrauma/abstract.00005373-200111000-00017.htm

J Invest Dermatol. 1988 Nov;91(5):440-5.

http://ajpcell.physiology.org/cgi/content/full/277/2/C320

Spicy V Burger

2 vegetarian burgers, cut into bite-sized pieces
1 red bell pepper, cut into bite-sized pieces
3 teaspoons paprika
1 teaspoon turmeric
1 teaspoon coarse ground black pepper
2 tablespoon freeze-dried chives
2 tablespoon canola oil

Preheat oiled frying pan, medium heat. Mix vegetarian burger and spices in a bowl. Add red bell pepper. Mix. Pour into frying pan. Stir mixture. Cook for 15 minutes. Serve.

Yield: serves two.

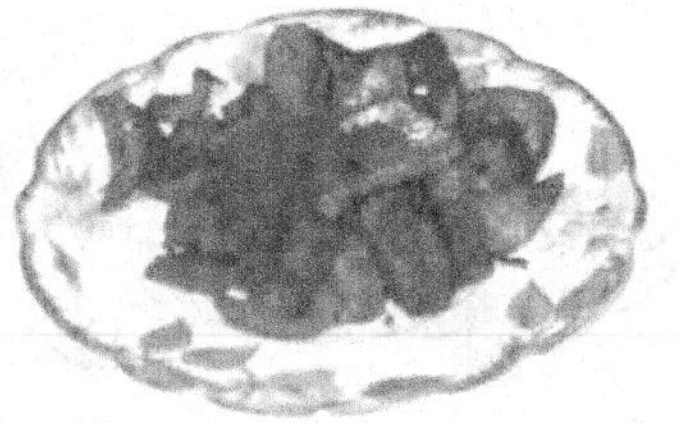

Wound

Multitude of reasons.

Injured? Take a multivitamin that contains vitamins A, C, and E; and zinc. These nutrients help wounds heal.

Here's the science:

Vitamin A supplementation improves the healing of wounds by activating a growth factor at the wound site.

Vitamin C is needed for collagen synthesis. Collagen is part of the extracellular matrix – the stuff between the cells.

Vitamin C is also an antioxidant. It helps protect tissue from the oxidative stresses involved in wound healing.

Vitamin E supplementation helps the wound make more of another growth factor that stimulates the synthesis of extracellular matrix.

Vitamin E is also an antioxidant.

Zinc deficiency is common. Zinc is needed to make Zinc-finger proteins. Zinc-finger proteins grab a hold of genetic switches and modulate the expression of genes, including genes for growth factors involved in healing.

---

http://www.pedresearch.org/cgi/content/abstract/55/6/935
J Invest Dermatol. 1988 Nov;91(5):440-5.
J Dermatol Sci. 1996 Mar;11(3):250-3.
http://springerlink.metapress.com/app/home/contribution.asp?wasp=agxy6ymhxr4uthg4wr8x&referrer=parent&backto=issue,14,14;journal,28,56;linkingpublicationresults,1:101491,1
J Int Med Res. 2003 Jan-Feb;31(1):26-30.
Kulak Burun Bogaz Ihtis Derg. 2003 Mar;10(3):87-92.
http://circres.ahajournals.org/cgi/content/full/92/1/104
Gen Pharmacol. 1998 Mar;30(3):423-7.
Int J Mol Med. 1999 Dec;4(6):615-20.
Int J Mol Med. 2001 Oct;8(4):433-8.
Nutrition. 1995 Jan-Feb;11(1 Suppl):93-9.
Acta Orthop Belg. 2003 Dec;69(6):546-51.

Wound

Aloe – all right.

Aloe aids wound healing when used either as a dressing for wounds or when the injured person drinks aloe juice ($^1/_2$ teaspoon).

Here's the science:

Aloe soothes minor burns.

Aloe enhances extracellular matrix formation at wound sites.

Early in the healing process, the stuff between the cells is largely composed of glycosaminoglycans (GAGs). Aloe stimulates the production of GAGs.

Aloe also enhances collagen synthesis. Collagen, another component of the extracellular matrix, helps give tissue its strength.

Aloe enhances cell proliferation at wound sites, which in turn promotes healing.

Clin Hemorheol Microcirc. 2003;29(3-4):239-46.
J Ethnopharmacol. 1998 Jan;59(3):179-86.
Mol Cell Biochem. 1998 Apr;181(1-2):71-6.
http://www.blackwell-synergy.com/openurl?genre=article&sid=nlm:pubmed&issn=0007-0963&date=2001&volume=145&issue=4&spage=535
J Am Podiatr Med Assoc. 1989 Nov;79(11):559-62.

21st Century Life

Pollution

Turn to turmeric

Scientists have found that mice living in polluted urban areas have more mutations. Well, if pollution is bad for rodents, what about us people?

After testing ancient bones, researchers have found that Southwest American Indians who lived 700-1000 years ago had a lead load one-thousandth of what adult Americans carry today. We didn't evolve to carry as much lead as we currently do. Even "modest" levels of lead exposure can result in psychiatric symptoms in adults and learning problems in children.

What can you do? One surprising answer is to use the spice turmeric.

Here's the science:

Curcumin, the active ingredient in turmeric, protects human DNA from chemical – benzo(a)pyrene – damage. DNA damage can lead to cancer.

Curcumin shields your brain from lead pollution. Research on rats found that curcumin significantly curtailed lead-induced brain damage.

---

http://www.sciencedirect.com/science?_ob=ArticleURL&_udi=B6VB5-3VWFXHR-D&_coverDate=12%2F31%2F1996&_alid=176295901&_rdoc=1&_fmt=&_orig=search&_qd=1&_cdi=5917&_sort=d&view=c&_acct=C000050221&_version=1&_urlVersion=0&_userid=10&md5=7a9e683a96bc6606c5856dcc4d206335
http://www.sciencedirect.com/science?_ob=ArticleURL&_udi=B6TGG-4B4S3CR-1&_coverDate=02%2F29%2F2004&_alid=168589785&_rdoc=1&_fmt=&_orig=search&_qd=1&_cdi=5254&_sort=d&view=c&_acct=C000050221&_version=1&_urlVersion=0&_userid=10&md5=7cba154e2158f64fe5655a10e71a7801
Sci Total Environ. 1991 Sep;107:205-36.
Mutat Res. 2004 Feb 14;557(2):203-13
J Occup Environ Med. 2003 Nov;45(11):1144-51.
http://www.eurekalert.org/pub_releases/2003-04/nioe-vll041503.php

21st Century Life

An apple a day keeps mercury at bay.

Mercury is toxic to the brain and heart. Industrial pollution has spewed mercury into our environment for centuries. Reducing sources of mercury pollution in our communities is important but doesn't completely solve the problem. Mercury pollution from decades and centuries past lingers in the environment. In addition, mercury released into the atmosphere can travel half-way around the world. Industrial emissions from developing countries, with fewer pollution controls, rain down on us. For example, China is a major source of mercury pollution in the western United States.

What can you do to help yourself and your family? Eat one or more pieces of fruit a day.

Here's the science:

Fruit lowers mercury levels. In a population study of Brazilians who ate a lot of fish (a source of mercury), those who also ate more fruit had lower mercury levels. Researchers speculate that the fruit fiber or phytochemicals might affect absorption or excretion of mercury.

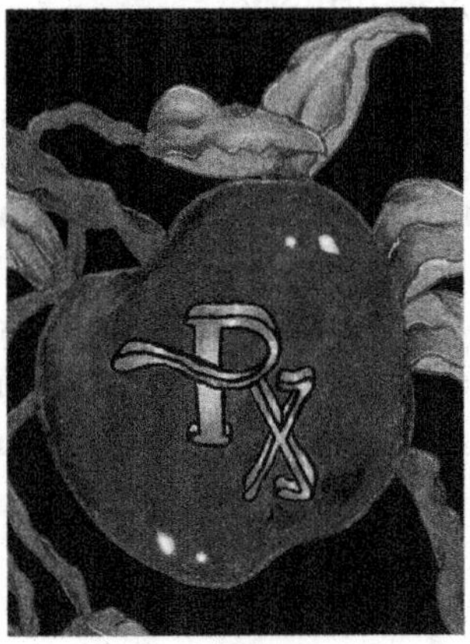

---

http://www.eurekalert.org/pub_releases/2002-12/uoc--mic121902.php
http://www.eurekalert.org/pub_releases/2002-11/jhub-maw112202.php
http://www.eurekalert.org/pub_releases/2003-06/ns-esm061103.php
http://www.sciencedirect.com/science?_ob=ArticleURL&_udi=B6WDS-49F9HPP-2&_coverDate=10%2F31%2F2003&_alid=176220671&_rdoc=1&_fmt=&_orig=search&_qd=1&_cdi=6774&_sort=d&view=c&_acct=C000050221&_version=1&_urlVersion=0&_userid=10&md5=8fd7ff91f9ad2b9823017dbbe465ab37

Don't be a fish out of water. Catch your breath.

Air pollution hits people with asthma the hardest. You can use an air purifier to improve the quality of air in your home; but do you want to be confined there? If you have asthma and want to breathe easier, take fish oil supplements. The omega-3 fatty acids found in fish oil may prevent or reduce asthma. If you suffer from asthma, take ten capsules of pharmaceutical-grade fish oil a day. Also, cut down on your consumption of oils that are rich in omega-6 fatty acids (corn, sunflower seed, safflower seed, cottonseed, and soybean).

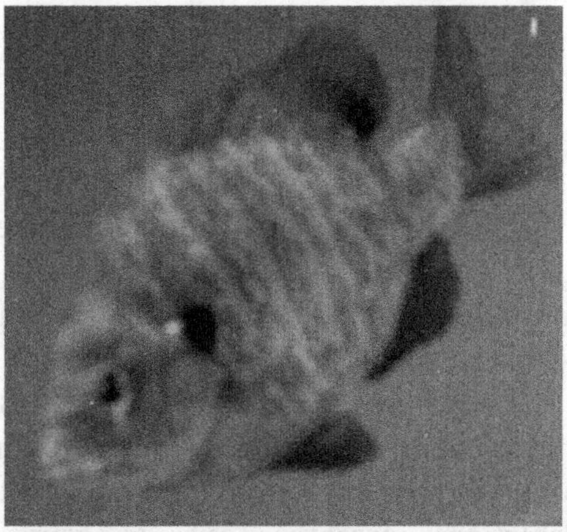

Here's the science:

Omega-3 fatty acids are anti-inflammatory. Inflammatory eicosanoids, which are made from omega-6 fatty acids, mediate asthma. A better ratio of omega-3 fatty acids (fish oil) to omega-6 fatty acids curbs the inflammatory response.

---

http://www.eurekalert.org/pub_releases/1999-09/UoSC-Aphc-100999.php
http://www.eurekalert.org/pub_releases/2004-05/ats-est052404.php
http://www.mja.com.au/public/issues/177_06_160902/mel10238_fm.html

21st Century Life

Ozone Depletion

Get a selenium shield.

The ozone layer reduces the level of DNA-damaging UV light that hits the earth. However, chemical pollution has depleted the ozone layer.

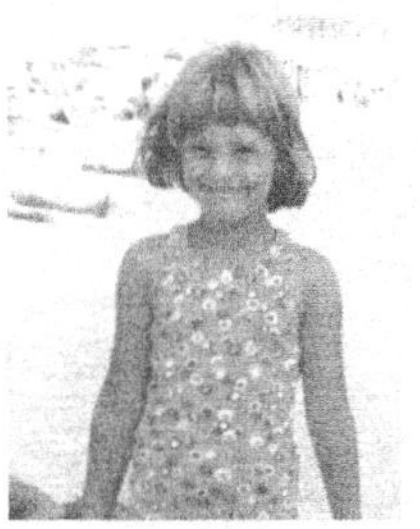

What can you do to protect yourself today? Take a multivitamin supplement containing selenium, and use sunscreen.

Here's the science:

Selenium supplementation reduces UV-induced cancer. In mice, selenium supplementation decreases tumor formation from UV exposure. In cell culture experiments, selenium decreases cell death from UV exposure by 71%.

The average person gets only 40% of the recommended allowance of selenium. Taking selenium supplementation is becoming more important as ozone depletion increases our exposure to harmful UV light.

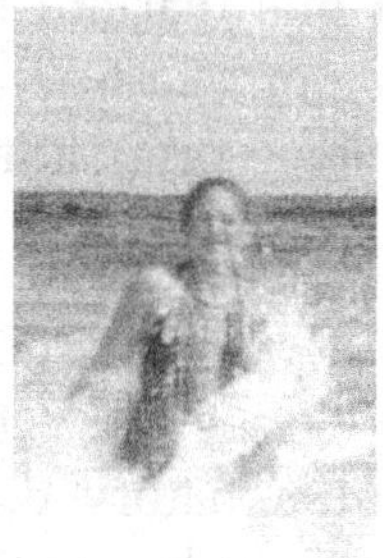

However, selenium shields the genome from only one of the ways UV light attacks DNA – oxidative damage from UV-generated free radicals. It does not guard against another form of UV-induced DNA damage, *photodimerization* – a knotting up of adjacent DNA bases. So keep your sunscreen on as well.

---

http://www.eurekalert.org/pub_releases/1999-03/CA-MSTO-040399.php
http://www.blackwell-synergy.com/openurl?genre=article&sid=nlm:pubmed&issn=0307-6938&date=2003&volume=28&issue=3&spage=294
http://www.blackwell-synergy.com/openurl?genre=article&sid=nlm:pubmed&issn=0007-0963&date=2003&volume=148&issue=5&spage=1001
http://www.biochemj.org/bj/332/0231/bj3320231.htm
http://www.eurekalert.org/pub_releases/1999-06/NOaA-Psrs-230699.php

21st Century Life

Terrorism

Be prepared to kick butt.

9/11/01. During the 20th century, hijackers took planes to places such as Cuba. People were told to cooperate with the hijackers so no one would get hurt. All that changed one clear September day. The current crop of terrorists will stop at nothing in their quest to destroy Western civilization. However, few flights have air marshals and few pilots are armed. In the 21st century, it's the duty of every able-bodied person to be prepared to fight back against hijackers. Start training today. The better your skills are, the better your chances are of beating the terrorists – remember, they're training too.

Web sites with more information about the martial arts:

JUDO
http://www.usjf.com/
http://www.usjudo.org/
http://www.nitojudo.com/

RUSSIAN MARTIAL ARTS
http://www.russianmartialart.com/
http://www.systema-nc.com/

TAE KWON DO
http://www.itatkd.com/

KUNG FU
http://www.shaolin.nl/

KARATE
http://www.ska.org/

Sensei Katz instructs her students….

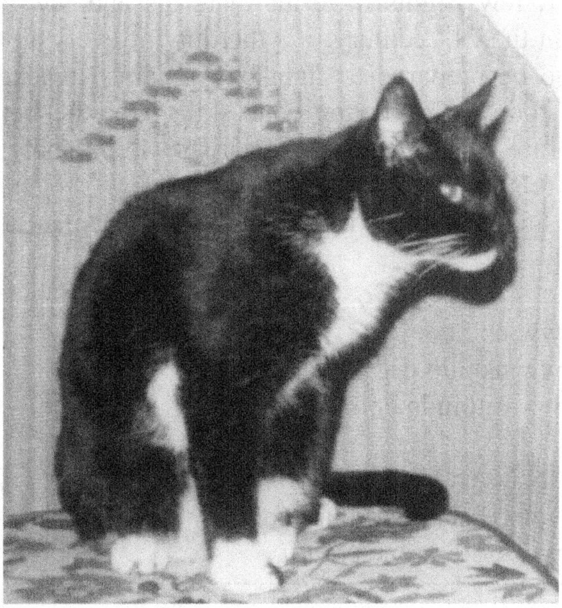

"Remember if you have to fight hijackers, it's claws *out* – shred those bastards."

Pantry shield.

In 1995, in a suburb of Detroit, a high school student created a primitive nuclear reactor in his mother's tool shed. The reactor spewed radiation, endangering area residents.

Not all geeks are Boy Scouts from the American middle class. Some may be among the ranks of terrorists. In the coming years, it's likely that terrorists will make radiological dirty bombs or even nuclear bombs.

If you are at ground zero of a nuclear bomb, there isn't much you can do. But what if you are on the edge of a nuclear event and exposed to low-to-moderate levels of radiation? How can you prepare for such a possibility? Keep a well-stocked pantry. You don't want to have to go to the store while fallout is raining down. To help shield yourself from the dangers of radiation, your pantry should include, among other foods: potassium iodide supplements, antioxidant supplements, turmeric supplements, juices, dried fruit such as raisins, tea bags and bottled water.

Here's the science:

Potassium iodide supplements provide iodine to out-compete radioactive iodine – from fallout – for a place in your thyroid. If radioactive iodine is allowed to take up residence in your thyroid, it can lead to cancer.

Antioxidants – radiation leads to free radical formation.

Vegetables, fruit, berries, and tea contain radioprotective phytochemicals.

Turmeric, taken orally, helps irradiated wounds to heal.

Ken Silverstein, The Radioactive Boy Scout: The True Story of a Boy and his Backyard Reactor, 2004.
J Environ Pathol Toxicol Oncol. 2004;23(2):145-51.
Indian J Exp Biol. 2001 Dec;39(12):1254-7.
J Exp Clin Cancer Res. 1998 Dec;17(4):431-4.
In Vivo. 2003 Mar-Apr;17(2):197-200.
J Surg Res. 2004 Jul;120(1):127-38.
Toxicology. 2003 Jul 15;189(1-2):1-20.

Be a bug-killing machine.

Authorities wouldn't know that a biological attack has taken place until people start falling over sick days later. However, most biological agents, such as small pox, don't have a 100% fatality rate. You can improve your odds by building a strong immune system now.

Practice Tai Chi or another form of moderate exercise.

Take a multivitamin with selenium and zinc.

Eat a balanced diet with plenty of fruits and vegetables. Eat eight or more servings of fruits and vegetables a day.

Take a pycnogenol supplement.

Here's the science:

Moderate physical activity, such as Tai Chi, enhances your resistance to infection. Exercise stimulates the release of immunostimulatory factors, which in turn activate various types of immune cells.

Selenium strengthens your immune system. Selenium deficiency makes you to be sicker if you get an infection.

Zinc boosts your defenses. Zinc stimulates your body's production of a protein called metallothionein. Metallothionein enhances your ability to fight infections.

Phytochemicals – plant chemicals – increase the responsiveness of immune cells.

Pycnogenol improves the immune cell function of elderly mice.

---

http://bjsm.bmjjournals.com/cgi/content/full/35/3/148
http://www.eurekalert.org/pub_releases/2002-09/tgso-nae093002.php
http://www.eurekalert.org/pub_releases/2003-11/aps-wfs111203.php
http://www.eurekalert.org/pub_releases/2001-04/UoNC-Sndc-2604101.php
http://www.eurekalert.org/pub_releases/1998-08/UoF-UoFR-060898.php
http://www.eurekalert.org/pub_releases/1999-04/CHRP-ZRCM-180499.php
J Nutr Biochem. 2003 Feb;14(2):90-8.
http://www.ajcn.org/cgi/content/abstract/68/1/164
Cell Mol Life Sci. 1998 Oct;54(10):1168-72.
http://www.ajcn.org/cgi/content/full/70/3/475S

21st Century Life

Eating plenty of vegetables is important for fighting off germs. The oregano in this recipe also has phytochemicals, which benefit the immune system.

Roasted Vegetables

2 red bell peppers
1 yellow squash
1 green squash
4 carrots
1 tablespoon balsamic vinegar
3 tablespoons canola oil
2 teaspoons oregano
¼ teaspoon salt
1 teaspoon coarse ground black pepper

Preheat oven to 400 degrees. Cut vegetables into bite-sized chucks. Place vegetables in large mixing bowl. Add balsamic vinegar. Toss well until vegetables absorb vinegar. Add other ingredients and toss. Pour mixture into a non-stick, roasting pan and spread out. Roast for about 25 minutes, stirring occasionally.

Yield: serves three.

Tijdschr Diergeneeskd. 2004 Mar 15; 129(6):178-81

21st Century Life

Here's another way to strengthen your immune system by adding a colorful vegetable to your diet.

Roasted Yams

2 yams
2 tablespoons balsamic vinegar
2 tablespoons canola oil
1 tablespoon oregano

Preheat oven to 350 degrees. Cut yams in half length-wise and place in a non-stick roasting pan. Drizzle balsamic vinegar on yams. Drizzle oil on yams. Sprinkle oregano on yams. Roast for about 35 – 40 minutes, until soft.

Yield: serves four.

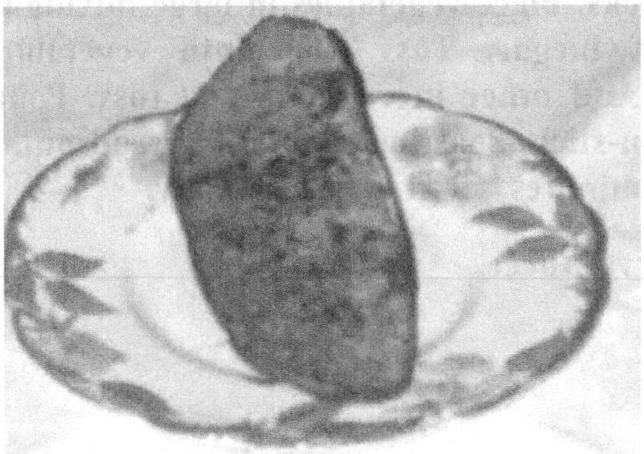

Still another way to get your veggies and build your immune system….

<u>Peppers Stuffed with Salad</u>

3 large red bell peppers
1 cup diced tomato
1 cup diced cucumber
½ cup diced red onion
1 cup feta cheese crumbles
2 tablespoons fresh oregano leaves
Extra-virgin olive oil, to taste
Balsamic vinegar, to taste

Toss tomatoes, cucumbers, onion, and feta cheese crumbles in a bowl. Add oregano leaves. Drizzle olive oil and vinegar on the salad. Toss. Cut bell peppers length-wise and deseed them. Scoop salad into bell peppers. Serve.

Yield: serves 6.

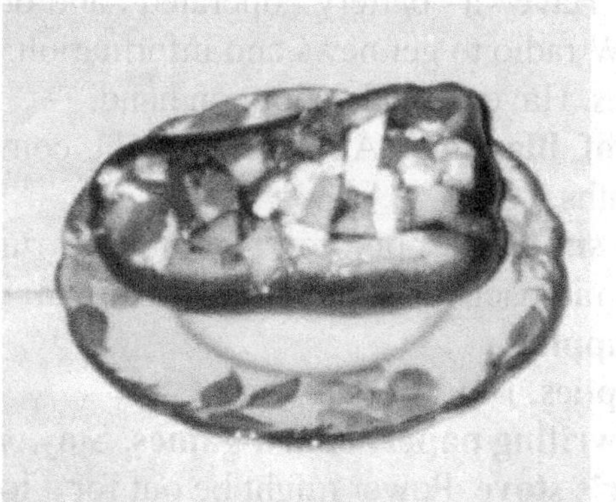

Home base – make your home your refuge of safety.

Cash. A cyber-attack or power failure could knockout ATM machines.

First aid kit. Include bandages, sterile gauze pads, adhesive tape, anti-microbial ointment, tea tree oil antiseptic, rubbing alcohol, aloe vera gel, pain medication, decongestant, turmeric supplements, potassium iodide supplements, anti-microbial mouthwash, and zinc lozenges.

Bottled water. A gallon a day per person for drinking plus extra for sponge baths.

Food. Rotate your pantry items to keep them fresh. Include items such as protein powder, fruit juice, dried fruit, canned foods, oatmeal, nuts, tea bags, multivitamins, etc.

Hand-crank can-opener. If the electricity is out, you can't use an electric one.

Power outage lights. They turn on when the power goes out. Otherwise you'll have to hunt for a flashlight in the dark.

Flashlights.

Radio. Have a battery operated and/or hand-crank AM/FM/SW radio to get news and information.

Batteries. Have a good supply on hand.

Plenty of blankets. An attack might come during the winter months.

Female supplies. You won't be able to run to the drug store while radioactive fallout is raining down.

Baby supplies.

Pet supplies. Don't forget Fluffy.

Books, writing paper, board games. Stay entertained.

Camper's stove. Power might be out for a long while.

Plastic trash bags for trash and to line the toilet if the water isn't running.

Also read http://www.chuckharder.com/blackout.htm

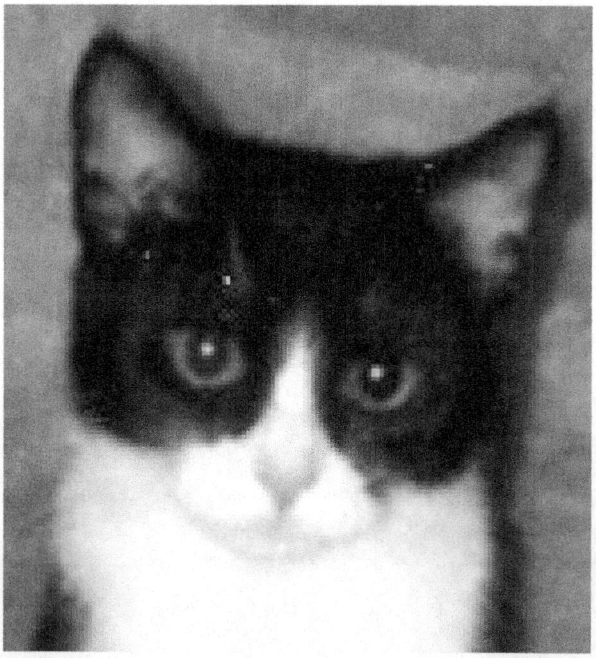

Don't let that bad-bad man Osama bin Laden hurt me – remember me when you get emergency supplies.

Author's Page

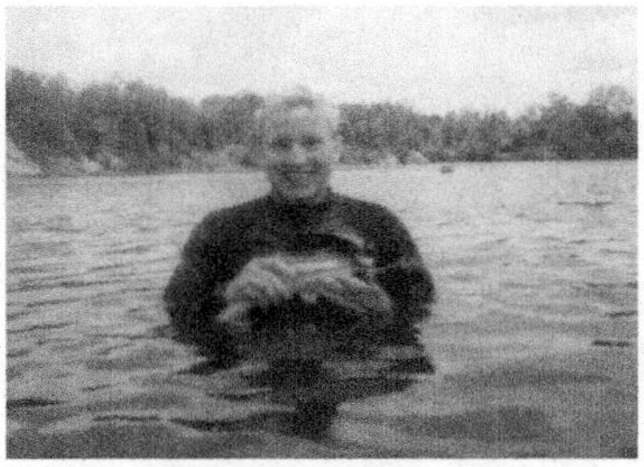

Celia Ross, M.S., is the author of technical pieces in biochemical and medical journals. She enjoys swimming laps at a local dive quarry and studying the martial arts.

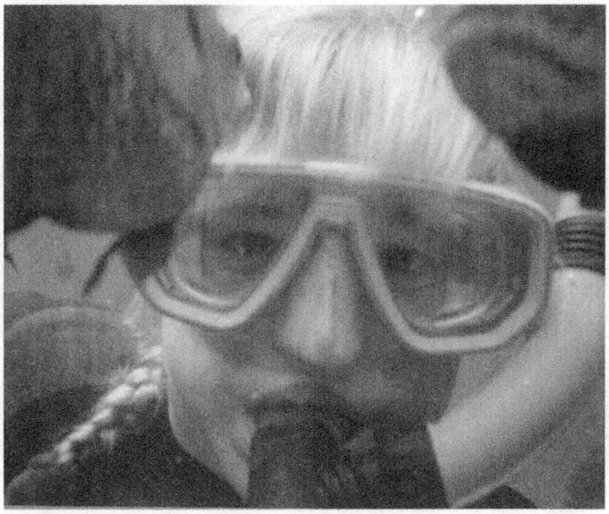

Visit my web site at

www.celiamross.com

celiamaryross@aol.com

Made in the USA
Monee, IL
13 September 2026

62977545R10070